# Advances in Psychosomatic Medicine

Vol. 11

Series Editor
*Thomas N. Wise*, Falls Church, Va.

Editors
*G. Fava*, Bologna; *H. Freyberger*, Hannover;
*F. Guggenheim*, Dallas, Tex.; *O.W. Hill*, London;
*Z.J. Lipowski*, Hanover, N.H.; *G. Lloyd*, Edinburgh;
*J.C. Nemiah*, Boston, Mass.; *P. Reich*, Boston, Mass.

Consulting Editors
*G.L. Engel*, Rochester, N.Y.; *H. Weiner*, Bronx, N.Y.
*L. Levi,* Stockholm

Editor Emeritus
*Franz Reichsman*, Brooklyn, N.Y.

S. Karger · Basel · München · Paris · London · New York · Sydney

# Consultation-Liaison throughout the World

Volume Editors
*Thomas N. Wise*, Falls Church, Va.
*Hellmuth Freyberger*, Hannover

6 figures and 14 tables, 1983

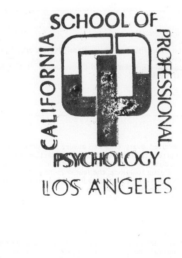

S. Karger · Basel · München · Paris · London · New York · Sydney

# Advances in Psychosomatic Medicine

Vol. 8: Psychosocial Aspects of Physical Illness
Lipowski, Z.J., Hanover, N.H. (ed.)
XIV+278 p., 17 fig., 4 tab., hard cover, 1972. ISBN 3-8055-1339-9

Vol. 9: Epidemiologic Studies in Psychosomatic Medicine
Kasl, S., New Haven, Conn., and Reichsman, F., Brooklyn, N.Y. (eds.)
X+226 p., 8 fig., 6 tab., hard cover, 1977. ISBN 3-8055-2654-7

Vol. 10: Psychotherapeutic Interventions in Life-Threatening Illness
Freyberger, H., Hannover (ed.)
XVIII+206 p., 2 fig., hard cover, 1980. ISBN 3-8055-3066-8

National Library of Medicine, Cataloging in Publication
Consultation-liaison throughout the world/
volume editors, Thomas N. Wise, Hellmuth Freyberger. -- Basel; New York: Karger, 1983.
(Advances in psychosomatic medicine; v. 11)
1. Psychiatry  2. Psychosomatic Medicine  3. Referral and Consultation  I. Freyberger, Hellmuth
II. Wise, Thomas Nathan, 1948–  III. Series
W1 AD81 v. 11  [WM 64 C758]
ISBN 3-8055-3667-4

Drug Dosage
The author and the publisher have exerted every effort to ensure that drug selection and dosage set forth in this text are in accord with current recommendations and practice at the time of publication. However, in view of ongoing research, changes in government regulations, and the constant flow of information relating to drug therapy and drug reactions, the reader is urged to check the package insert for each drug for any change in indications and dosage and for added warnings and precautions. This is particularly important when the recommended agent is a new and/or infrequently employed drug.

# Contents

Contents

## Summary View

# In memoriam
# Prof. Dr. med. Arthur Jores
*10. 2. 1901 – 11. 9. 1982*

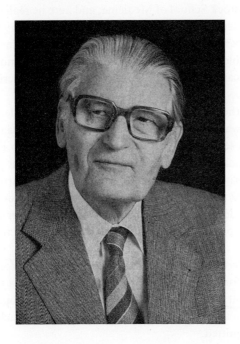

*Arthur Jores*, Professor emeritus and formerly Director, Second Department of Medicine, Eppendorf Hospital, University of Hamburg, died on November 9, 1982 at the age of 81 years after 8 months of serious illness in which his wife *Hanna* supported him with much loving care and patience.

*Jores* may be regarded as one of the most brilliant and original figures of German internal medicine. In his person, an engaged doctor's attitude and excellent rhetoric and didactic abilities were combined with imperturbable provocative verbal power and consequent research activities. This combination of attitudes helped *Jores* in his decision to start his great pioneer work in psychosomatic medicine.

Starting from his time at the Department of Medicine, General Hospital Hamburg-Altona, *Jores'* career was decisively influenced by his teacher, Dr. *Leopold Lichtwitz*. *Lichtwitz* opened to *Jores* the field of both medicine and, particularly, biological rhythmus research and endocrinology. Initially *Jores* was firmly convinced that *Lichtwitz* would be offered a chair and that he could accompany him. But, *Lichtwitz* as a Jew was obliged to emigrate to the United States.

Now, *Jores* moved to Dr. *Hans Curschmann*, Chairman and Professor of Medicine, University of Rostock School of Medicine, and here he realized his 'Habilitation' with the consequent nomination as 'Privatdozent' in 1934. His habilitation included experimental work with regard to the melanophoric hormone. *Jores* was able to prove that the melanophoric hormone is an autonomous one which can be separated from the remaining anterior pituitary hormones.

In this Rostock position, the professionally hopeful career was suddenly interrupted in 1936 when he was denounced by a colleague. The colleague had discovered, in the clinic's secretariat, post from *Jores* addressed to Dr. *Lichtwitz* and in which he included his own book entitled *Medicine for dentists*, with reprints and private dedications. Then, *Jores* was warned effectively by a Nazi follower to avoid contact with *Lichtwitz*. However, *Jores* decidedly rejected this demand, was forced to leave the university and found temporarily a new place of work in the pharmaceutical factory 'Promonta' in Hamburg.

*Jores* was forced to suffer a further humiliation in the Second World War when he was remanded for a period of 6 months. This arrest was the consequence of *Jores'* statement, following the heavy air raids on Hamburg, that we would be obliged to do all we could to prevent this 'cruel spectacle'. In spring 1944, *Jores* was acquitted.

Following his very distinguished and well-known predecessors, Drs. *Schottmüller* and *Weitz*, *Jores* was offered a chair of medicine at the University of Hamburg School of Medicine, in autumn 1945 and nominated as director of the Second Department of Medicine, Eppendorf Hospital. The position as rector of the University of Hamburg was filled by *Jores* in 1953. In 1958, *Jores* refused the nomination to become chairman and professor of medicine, University of Munich.

Following his nomination in Hamburg, *Jores* was initially concerned with building up his clinic as a center of endocrinology by gaining talented co-workers and by the institutionalization of laboratories. But soon, *Jores* delegated these activities to his endocrinological co-workers and started his intensive work in the field of psychosomatic medicine which he consequently performed up to his retirement in 1967. In his *Selbstdarstellung (Self-portrait) Jores* [Quoted from: Arthur Jores; in Pongratz, Psychotherapie in Selbstdarstellungen (psychotherapy in self-portraits) (Huber, Bern 1973)] writes that earlier he had been asked repeatedly why he did not remain in his former research topic endocrinology, but set foot on 'the highly problematic and still staggering ground of psychological medicine'. Then, his regular answer was: 'I was obliged to do it by my patients.'

The central point of *Jores*' psychosomatical-psychotherapeutical concept was the term 'specifically human disease'. On this basis, *Jores* relates the medical fields of psychosomatics, neurosis theory and psychotherapy to an anthropology in which man and animal are differentiated systematically. In *Jores*' anthropology, a multiplicity of possibilities regarding development makes it a task to deal with this development and, vice versa, the marked developmental impairments mean a psychotherapeutic task too. On this basis, *Jores* inaugurated a special variant of psychotherapeutic counselling and psychotherapeutic consultation.

Besides his personal anthropological view, *Jores* was distinguished by carefully directed clinico-psychosomatical interventions (including their description) vis-à-vis psychosomatic patients and those organically ill patients with marked secondary-psychic alterations who were suffering from severe diseases. Furthermore, and in spite of his anthropological view, *Jores was* very concerned to gain as co-workers psychoanalytically oriented doctors and psychologists within the framework of his clinico-psychosomatical section. For *Jores* perceived increasingly that psychoanalysis represented both the central theory with regard to the explanation of psychodynamic processes in psychosomatic patients and the optimal treatment possibility if we also include the modifications of psychoanalytic therapy, e.g. supportive psychotherapy with superficial confrontation and interpretation work. Finally and within the framework of his lectures to students, *Jores* systematically organized psychosomatical arrangements at a time when these arrangements occurred extremely rarely in the medical faculties of West Germany.

Starting from *Jores*' extensively dynamic activities, not only a Jores school of internists, but also one of psychosomaticists exists. This combination of medicine and psychosomatics has impressively precipitated itself in *Jores*' thematically extraordinarily multifarious publication index. On the basis of this index, such an unusually large number of scientific contributions and monographs is evident that they cannot be presented here in detail.

Following 1945, *Jores* was able to realize his high talent as a pioneer and to bear all those disappointments and failures which are customary for the pioneer specifically with regard to the psychosomatical movement. But in spite of these disappointments, which were particularly provoked by the rigid acting-out of highly conservative German psychiatrists, *Jores* adhered firmly and imperturbably to the psychosomatic movement. Especially, the violent antipsychoanalytical resistance of very orthodox German psychiatrists in the fifties and in the first half of the sixties represented the main reason for the fact that in West Germany, following the Second World War, clinical psychosomatics was not developed in psychiatry but in clinico-medical settings (see the West German chapter 'Introduction' in this volume).

A long time (1977) after his retirement, *Jores*, together with his colleagues, acted as the editor of the textbook entitled *Praktische Psychosomatik (Practice in Psychosomatics)*, which sold a very high number of copies and has recently appeared in its second edition.

Sadly, *Jores* was not to experience, together with a lot of German and foreign colleagues, by whom he was highly admired, the coming Hamburg World Congress of Psychosomatics (International College of Psychosomatic Medicine) which is arranged by 'his' Department of Psychosomatics, Center of Medicine, Eppendorf University Hospital, under the chairmanship of his pupils, Dr. Dr. *Adolf-Ernst Meyer* and Dr. *Hubert Speidel*, and will take place in July 1983. This coming World Congress, which highlights the international relevance of psychosomatics in West Germany, would not have been realized with regard to organization and themes structure without the so highly effective pioneer work of *Jores*.

Besides his pioneer work with regard to psychosomatic medicine in Germany, *Jores* was one of the founders of our series entitled *Advances in Psychosomatic Medicine*. Together with Drs. *Felix Deutsch* (Boston, USA) and *Berthold Stokvis* (Leyden, The Netherlands), *Jores* began his editorial work in 1959. The present editorial board highly appreciates the past editorial work of these three senior citizens, colleagues and fatherly friends.

*H. Freyberger*, Hannover

# Dedication

This volume is dedicated to Prof. *Franz Reichsman*, Professor of Medicine (in Psychiatry), State University of New York, Downstate Medical Center. As Editor-in-Chief of *Advances in Psychosomatic Medicine* for the past decade, Dr. *Reichsman* has provided unparalleled leadership in developing the *Advances*. He continues to set an example in clinical acumen, educational ability and critical thinking so that all of us may have a model of excellence to which we strive.

# Introduction

Consultation-liaison psychiatry is a clinical discipline. In contradistinction to psychosomatic or psychophysiologic, terms which connote causality, consultation-liaison activities are the actual clinical derivatives of situations where psychological, biological and social issues interact. General hospital psychiatrists who perform psychiatric consultations, internists interested in psychosocial factors, and behavioral psychologists focusing upon psychophysiology all contribute to such activities. In the United States there has been a tremendous growth of this biopsychosocial intervention. Generous government funding and psychiatry's reapproachment to medicine have fostered this process. To date, most reports of consultation-liaison activities have been limited to work within the United States. This volume attempts to fill that void by reporting upon consultation-liaison endeavors throughout the world. Contributors were selected to discuss the growth of consultation-liaison activities in their respective countries. Unfortunately, colleagues from Australia, Africa as well as Asia were unable to contribute.

The volume is organized into three sections. The introductory section outlines the history and scope of consultation-liaison activities. This section provides a background to psychosomatic medicine as well as the applied discipline of consultation-liaison psychiatry and liaison medicine. Dr. *Hoyle Leigh* summarizes the history of psychosomatic medicine and its evolution into the clinical areas of consultation liaison work. Dr. *Donald Oken* reviews the growth of liaison medicine and consultative psychiatry focusing upon organizational formats, clinical tasks and financial realities that limit growth of the discipline. Dr. *Daniel Schubert's* chapter utilizes a dialectic paradigm to consider the practical differences and similarities between consultation psychiatry and liaison medicine.

The second section consists of contributors from various parts of the world who describe consultation-liaison activities in their country. Each of these contributors was given the following statement:

'Liaison medicine is a discipline wherein the liaison worker becomes part of the department, team or unit. He is a psychosocial expert but preferably has a background in the discipline in which he will work, i.e. medicine, pediatrics, obstetrics, etc. If the liaison worker is a psychiatrist, it is accepted that he will acquire knowledge and skills within this department in addition to the psychosocial expertise. In contradistinction, consultative psychiatry implies that a psychiatrist's function is either as time-limited, episodic visitor doing consultation or engaging in a more longitudinal process within a department, team or unit. The major difference between medicine and consultative psychiatry is that in consultative psychiatry there is a clear identification of the physician as a psychiatrist. He is just that – a physician trained in psychiatry whereas the liaison worker functions in a more overlapping role. Although these definitions are more clearly polarized, there obviously exists a continuum. The role of the psychosomaticist, if such an individual exists, also functions within this continuum. Because the term psychosomatics implies causality, I have chosen not to define it as such. More recent work tends to emphasize psychosocial variables which correlate with physical illness or medical service utilization und thus transcends the traditional psychosomatic search for causal factors.

With these definitions in mind, each contributor was asked to discuss the history and development of liaison medicine and consultative psychiatry within their respective countries as well as a discussion of any 'psychosomatic movement' that had developed. Specific activities within each department as well as how such consultative activities fit into the unique characteristics of the country's health delivery system were to be delineated. Educational programs were to be described; in particular, the role of consultative and liaison services in augmenting psychosocial knowledge, awareness and expertise; finally, research activities that were presently underway and the future of consultation activities were to be reported.

Thus, Dr. *Sabonge* and colleagues described their activities in Panama. Dr. *Ryn* reviewed similar activities in the Eastern European country of Poland. Dr. *Avni* reports upon consultation-liaison psychiatry in Israel. Dr. *Gath* and Dr. *Mayou* discuss their own specific work in consultation-liaison psychiatry in Great Britain. Dr. *Ishikawa* reports on psychosomatic medicine in Japan, while Dr. *Fava* discusses consultation-liaison psychiatry in Italy. Other Western European contributors include psychosomatic leaders as Drs. *Askevold* and *Pierloot*, who discuss their activities in Norway and Belgium, respectively. The section on clinical contributions is completed by a comprehensive review on liaison activities in West Germany. The scope and breadth of this chapter reflects the energy and endeavors of West German psychosomaticists who have developed their own model which appears highly effective within the German health care system. The development of independent departments of psychosomatics with a close relationship to medicine appears unique in its organizational format. By organization of categorical departments with their own inpatient units, the West German model has flourished. The final section is that of a summarizing chapter by Dr. *Geoffrey Lloyd*, who has already contributed an important perspective on an international view of consultation-liaison psychiatry [*Lloyd*, 1980].

The volume gives a varied picture of consultation-liaison psychiatry developments throughout the world. Such activities take great energy as they require demarcation from parent subspecialties whether they be psychiatry or medicine. Organized professional societies of either psychiatrists or internists may not understand the role of the psychosomaticist. Recurrent themes appear throughout the volume which may be summarized as follows: Fiscal limitations exist in such interface activities. Traditional 'turf' issues also arise. The success of liaison activities depends on the comfort of the culture of the medical setting and health delivery system with the team concept, i.e. sharing various responsibilities and expertise to deliver the best health care. Finally, many of the contributors appear optimistic about the future of their work. Thus, the gradient of the endeavor appears to be uphill but the momentum is increasing and the friction diminishing. It is hoped that this volume will allow new information about the role of consultation-liaison endeavors and psychosomatics from an international perspective. By looking at problems both unique and common to various countries, solutions may be found to the impediments in delivering medical care that addresses both biologic, psychological and social parameters. This is a modest attempt to better understand how to adopt a new biopsychosocial approach that *Engel* [1977] has urged.

The editors would like to gratefully acknowledge the ongoing help and support of Prof. *Franz Reichsman*, who helped develop the idea for such a volume. Drs. *Oscar Hill, John Nemiah, Z.J. Lipowski, Milton Rosenbaum, L. Levi*, and *P. Sainsbury* all provided critical reviews and suggestions. It is obvious that each one of the contributors must be personally thanked to take the time out from their already busy schedules to contribute to such a volume. The organization and production of this volume could not have been possible without the invaluable efforts of Mrs. *Anne H. Hill* who worked many hours on the manuscripts.

*References*

Engel, G.L.: The need for a new medical model: a challenge for biomedicine. Science
    *196:* 129–135 (1977).
Lloyd, G.G.: Liaison psychiatry from a British perspective. Gen. Hosp. Psychiat. *2:* 46–51
    (1980).

*Thomas N. Wise,*
Editor-in-Chief

# Theoretical Aspects

Adv. psychosom. Med., vol. 11, pp. 1–22 (Karger, Basel 1983)

## The Evolution of Psychosomatic Medicine and Consultation-Liaison Psychiatry [1, 2]

*Hoyle Leigh*

Yale University School of Medicine, Division of Psychiatric Consultation-Liaison and Outpatient Services, Yale-New Haven Hospital, Yale Behavioral Medicine Clinic, New Haven, Conn., USA

### Introduction

In ancient times, there was little distinction between physical and mental diseases, both believed to be caused by gods and evil spirits. Both spiritual (shamanistic rites) and physical (e.g. trephination to let the evil spirit out) treatments were used for all disorders [*Sigerist*, 1951]. This holism of body and mind (with emphasis on the spirit causing physical disease) seems to have been prevalent in many parts of the world, including the Egyptian, Babylonian, Hindu and Chinese ancient cultures.

*Hippocrates* (460–370 BC) was the first physician to integrate physiology, psychology, and anatomy (of his day, to be sure) to explain disorders. For example, he believed madness to be caused by excessive bile; hysteria, by wandering uterus (he believed marriage to be the best cure for this condition); and that profound emotional states could affect the color of skin of unborn children [*Zilboorg*, 1967].

*Hippocrates* believed that disease was caused not by spirits, but by an imbalance of body fluids; blood, mucus, black bile, and yellow bile. Further, the imbalance could be caused by a similar imbalance in the patient's environment. He warned the visiting physician to consider the attitude, wind direction, purity of water supply, and season of the year before making any diagnosis [*Kaplan*, 1980]. *Hippocrates* wrote, 'in order to cure the human body, it is necessary to have a knowledge of the whole of things' [*Dunbar*, 1954].

[1] Supported in part by USPHS Grant MH 13793.

[2] Portions of this article were published in Leigh H. and Reiser M.F.: Major trends in psychosomatic medicine. The psychiatrist's evolving role in medicine. Ann. intern. Med. *87:* 233–239 (1977). Reprinted with permission.

*Galen* (130–200 AD), physician of emperor *Marcus Aurelius*, systematized medical knowledge of the Roman era through the integration of Hippocratic tradition with his own observations. He placed particular importance on the brain as the seat of rational soul (the heart and the liver were believed to be the seats of two irrational souls). He further believed that the seat of the soul is inseparable from the nerve centers [*Zilboorg*, 1967].

The physiologic unitarianism of *Hippocrates* and *Galen* was replaced by another, an irrational type, with the advent of the dark ages. During the middle ages, sin was considered to be the etiology of all diseases and demonic possession was thought to be particularly responsible for serious mental illnesses.

A revival in interest in nature and the human body during the renaissance (16th to 18th centuries) together with the invention of scientific instruments such as the telescope and the microscope, paved the way for the development of scientific medicine. *René Descartes* (1596–1650), the French mathematician and philosopher, was instrumental, to a large extent, in developing the philosophical foundations for the study of nature through his mind-matter dualism – by accepting the reality of both spirit and matter, and the application of reason as a tool of investigation. This dualism, on the other hand, relegated the study of the mind and emotions to philosophers and theologians, not to scientists.

This mind-body dualism has pervaded medicine despite the scientific efforts of such great physicians as *Pinel, Kraepelin,* and *Freud.* In fact, the psychodynamic elucidation of psychoneuroses by *Freud*, perhaps, contributed to this dualism by showing that some disorders have 'functional' causes. A frequently encountered example, familiar to most of us, is a physician requesting psychiatric consultation on a patient to determine whether the symptoms are 'functional', or to request transfer of the patient to the psychiatric unit because 'organic causes' have been ruled out.

The goal of this paper is to describe some salient features in the recent developments in psychosomatic medicine in the United States, which led to a redefinition of psychosomatic medicine as a comprehensive, holistic approach to all patients.

### Psychodynamic Investigations

In this line of investigation, psychoanalysts and psychoanalytically oriented physicians have focused attention on the possible role of psychodynamic conflicts in the origin of certain medical diseases, in studies that have largely paralleled the development of psychoanalysis in this country. As an example of this approach, we shall discuss *Alexander's* [1950] work briefly, although many other investigators have also made important contributions to this line of research [for other reviews of psychodynamic formulations see *Reiser*, 1975; *Lipowski*, 1968; *Kimball*, 1969].

*Alexander's* major works were done in the 1930s and 1940s in the Chicago Institute of Psychoanalysis. One of his major theoretical contributions was the differentiation between 'visceral neuroses' or psychosomatic disorders and 'conversion hysteria'. He made the distinction between conversion hysteria and psychosomatic disorders on the basis of the nervous system involved: somatosensory and special sensory nerves in the former, and the autonomic nervous system in the latter. In addition, he pointed out that actual tissue damage is present in psychosomatic disorders, whereas no tissue damage (except possible disuse atrophy) occurs in conversion hysteria.

*Alexander's* theory concerning the pathogenesis of 'psychosomatic disorders' was conflict-specific and was based on psychoanalytic investigations of patients with illnesses frequently observed to be related to psychologic stress and conflict. He theorized that specific unresolved psychologic conflicts were accompanied by prolonged specific autonomic arousal, representing the somatic concomitant of repressed and suppressed affects. For example, in the case of duodenal ulcer, he postulated that a life situation that activated conflicted longings for love would be accompanied by gastric overactivity and so contribute to duodenal ulceration in the presence of specific constitutional vulnerability. His investigations gave rise to the notion that psychologic factors played a major etiologic role in some diseases and that such diseases should be considered 'psychosomatic'.

This theoretical framework prompted treatment of these 'psychosomatic diseases' with psychotherapy or psychoanalysis. It also influenced the character of the psychosomatic services that were established in general hospitals. This 'psychosomatic approach' was practiced with almost the same kind of zeal that characterized psychiatry in general right after World War II. After peaking in the 1950s, it suffered a similar fate: the consequences of promising too much.

Inherent in this approach were certain methodologic and conceptual difficulties that arose chiefly because the data were based primarily on recollections of memories and associations during psychoanalysis. Almost everything we experience acquires symbolic psychic meanings. Thus, even physical symptoms can be meaningfully related to ongoing psychic life with its conflicts and needs, when investigated by psychoanalytic methods. This retrospective elucidation of meaning alone, however, could not clarify questions of proximal causation. Failure to recognize this fact often resulted in a premature closure of investigation into factors other than psychodynamic and psychosocial (for example, genetic, immunologic, infectious, or traumatic) that might contribute to the pathogenesis of an illness.

Current practice has now changed from the earlier notion that the presence of a 'psychosomatic disease' per se was adequate indication for psychotherapy. As for any medical patients, psychotherapy for patients with a 'psychosomatic disease' is indicated if the psychologic problems, in their own right, constitute valid reason for it. In the course of psychotherapy for cases in which psychological conflicts are activating pathophysiologic patterns, amelioration of the physical condition may occur as a consequence of reduced psychologic conflicts.

### Psychophysiologic and Psychosocial Investigations

This line of development is characterized by an empirical, experimental approach. In the early days, it focused on the effect of nonspecific stress on the organism. *Cannon's* work in the 1920s and 1930s concerning the fight-flight reaction is a good example. *Wolf and Wolff* [1947], contemporaries of *Alexander*, made important contributions by bringing psychiatric questions into the research laboratory and promoting the addition of the experimental method to clinical methods. They formulated adaptive, defensive psychophysiologic patterns, which might result in tissue damage and illness if prolonged. According to their theory, for example, the physiologic correlate of the psychologic defensive wish to get rid of an unpleasant idea might be associated with the hyperfunction of the organ for ejection-riddance – the colon – and resultant diarrhea.

Technologic developments of the past two decades ushered in a new blossoming of investigations along this experimental line. Such disciplines and methods as sophisticated biochemical assay techniques and computer science have brought about major developments in neurobiology and social sciences.

For example, in the classic psychosomatic diseases, such as peptic ulcer, it became possible to define and investigate the relation between constitutional or genetic vulnerability and psychosocial stress factors. *Weiner* et al. [1957] showed in the late 1950s that increased serum pepsinogen level, which is genetically determined, could be used as an indicator of vulnerability to peptic ulcer under conditions of a nonspecific stress like basic training in the army. In their study, those who developed peptic ulcer were found to have the personality configuration that followed *Alexander's* formulations. In addition and without exception, they also had constitutionally high serum pepsinogen levels, and the stress of basic training for them was such that activation of the specific conflict described by *Alexander* ensured. It is clear that predisposing constitutional factors are present in such other illnesses as hypertension or coronary disease. For a comprehensive review concerning various factors in the pathogenesis of the classic 'psychosomatic disorders', see *Weiner* [1977].

### Development of a 'Systems Model'

More recent experimental investigations have led to a change in the conceptual model of psychosomatic illness from a linear, multiple factor model to a nonlinear, interactional field or systems model. This model, which posits interactions between genetic 'givens' and the environment, postulates phenotypic expressions and mutual feedback in both somatic and behavioral spheres. According to this model, each individual's constitution includes genetic 'givens' as well as the results of early experience, and his development is influenced by multiple biologic and psychosocial factors in his bio-psychosocial environment. The mutual feedback between the behavioral and somatic dimensions and between the individual and his environment continue throughout his development and adult life.

For example, it can be postulated that the same genetic trait may be expressed phenotypically in an infant by high serum pepsinogen levels in the somatic sphere and high 'oral needs' in the behavioral-psychologic sphere. In the course of development and in interaction with significant others, such an individual would be likely to develop a psychologic conflict over 'oral dependency', and at a time of stress, the activation of the conflict might result in psychophysiologic consequences, which, given the existing vulnerability for peptic ulcer, might precipitate the disease. Once the disease developed, responses to the disease and its treatment, such as reactions to pain and hospitalization, might also affect its course.

This model clarifies the need to understand and evaluate all the major factors that might contribute to the pathogenesis of an illness and perpetuate it rather than attempting to isolate a single cause or a series of linear causal events.

It may be useful and proper to extrapolate from this model to a general systems approach to all medical illness (fig. 1). The general systems approach implies that multiple subsystems, such as constitutions and personality, determine the state of the individual system through constant mutual interaction and feedback. The individual, in turn, is a subsystem of the society, being in constant interaction and feedback with other individuals and groups within it. This approach emphasizes the interaction and feedback among a patient's somatic symptoms, behavior, and sociocultural milieu. For example, depression may be a behavioral symptom of a physical disease (for example, carcinoma of the tail of the pancreas). The depression may result in self-neglect and a tendency not to seek medical attention, thus allowing progression of the medical disease. If this model were applied to all medical illness, it would call for a comprehensive understanding of the various systems and their interactions, which would lead to judicious systems intervention as a part of treatment. A number of investigators have contributed to the development of a systems model, *Menninger* [1963] and *Engel* [1977] among others. We shall examine some of the important recent studies that have contributed to the development of this comprehensive approach.

## Behavioral Factors in Medical Illness

Established overt behavior patterns and psychologic states have been linked with certain physical illnesses. For example, *Friedman and Rosenman's* [1959, 1974] well-known 'coronary prone overt behavior pattern A' involves such characteristics as ambitiousness, hard-driving impatience, restlessness in individuals who always seem to function on a deadline basis, always with a sense of urgency [*Jenkins*, 1976]. It still remains to be seen, however, whether treatment of the overt behavior pattern A definitely results in a lowered risk of coronary disease. An alternative explanation of the correlation may be that the behavioral pattern and the vulnerability to coronary disease are both manifestations of the same constitutional trait.

Prospective studies have shown that individuals who have an elevation of the depression scale on the Minnesota Multiphasic Personality Inventory (MMPI) are more apt to develop myocardial infarction without preexisting angina pectoris [*Bruhn* et al., 1969], and also have a bad prognosis once myocardial infarction occurs. Patients undergoing open-heart surgery have a poor prognosis if depressed before surgery [*Kennedy and Bakst*, 1966; *Kimball*, 1969]. Although these studies show the correlation of preexisting

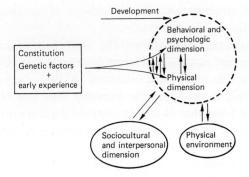

*Fig. 1.* Comprehensive model for all diseases.

psychologic states and morbidity, the data do not exclude the possibility that both the psychologic states and the physical manifestations might be a result of the same underlying process. Certainly, there are a number of disease processes that manifest behavioral disturbances before the specific organic symptoms appear. These include depression in occult neoplasms such as cancer of the tail of the pancreas, psychosis in pernicious anemia or lupus erythematosus, and many others.

### Role of Psychosocial Environment

While new investigations, starting in the late 1950s and continuing through the 1960s and 1970s, proved the importance of the constitutional factors in somatic illnesses, they also proved the importance of psychosocial environment in the development of a number of somatic illnesses. For example, *Henry* et al. [1971] were able to construct a psychosocial environment in which mice almost invariably developed hypertension, and another environment in which susceptible mice strains inevitably developed breast carcinoma [*Henry* et al., 1975]. The hypertension environment was created by constructing a cage system in which the animals were under constant threat of dominance challenge and had to compete for food in a territorial manner. The cancer environment involved a situation of forced breeding, in which the mice were kept in a constant state of readiness to reproduce, while the offspring were always removed after delivery. This resulted in a disorganization of the social structure and 100% incidence of mammary cancer in the susceptible strain female subjects.

Epidemiologic studies have repeatedly showed the significance of grief after bereavement as an important psychosocial factor favoring the development of somatic illnesses, such as myocardial infarction. A 1967 study in Wales [*Rees and Lutkins*, 1967] showed that the mortality after loss of a first-degree relative was seven times that of the age-matched control group. Interestingly, the relatives of those who died away from home had a mortality rate double that of those whose relatives died at home.

*Schmale* [1972] and *Engel and Schmale* [1967] have studied the psychologic states in which medical illnesses in general seemed to appear and hypothesized that a specific psychologic state, which they call the 'giving up-given up complex', provided an especially favorable setting for morbidity. This psychologic state, characterized by feelings of helplessness and hopelessness, is presumed to be associated with a physiologic state of conservation-withdrawal, with anabolic metabolic balance, in contradistinction to the fight-flight reaction with adrenal activation described by *Cannon*. Such 'permissive states' for the occurrence of somatic disorders may not be confined to conditions resembling depression and grief. Any type of life change, including change of residence, marriage, or even promotions, might contribute to a state of vulnerability to organic illness, according to the studies by *Rahe* [1972] and *Holmes and Rahe* [1968]. They were able to show, in a number of populations, that those individuals who had experience in a large number of life changes, good and bad, had a higher risk of developing almost any kind of physical illness. Death of spouse, however, was the highest ranking among the stressful events, having a value of 100 life change units.

A major question in psychosomatic medicine today is, what are the psychophysiologic states and mechanisms whereby, given the predisposition and favorable environment for development of disease, psychosocial events such as life changes or bereavement may actually trigger a disease?

*The Immune System – a Possible Mediating Mechanism*

A number of recent studies indicate that changes in the immune system, especially the T cell function, may occur under certain stressful situations, which may mediate the occurrence of disease [*Bartrop* et al., 1977; *Paclidis and Chirigos*, 1980; *Rogers* et al., 1979; *Stein* et al., 1976]. Immunologic changes may be secondary to changes in endocrine function (e.g. cortisol levels) in some cases, but may be directly related to autonomic discharges and central neurotransmitter activity in others in view of the fact that receptors for neurotransmitters have been demonstrated in lymphocytes.

### Biologic Rhythms

A related question concerns biologic rhythms and altered states of consciousness. For example, do certain illnesses occur in conjunction with the changes in autonomic and neuroendocrine reactivity that are associated with specific central nervous system states that occur in cycles, that is, at certain times of the day or month? Before the dawn of the present century, *Breuer and Freud* [1955] postulated that a 'hypnoidal state' might be associated with the development of hysterical symptoms. Psychosomatic theories, however, with few exceptions [*Reiser*, 1966; *Schur*, 1953, 1955], have not paid much attention to the possibility that distinct and definable central nervous system states may correlate with different states of consciousness as well as with altered physiologic reactivity that may be conducive or permissive to the development of disease. Rapid eye movement (REM) states, for example, occur every 90–120 min during sleep in man and are associated with vivid dreams and strong and variable physiologic arousal. Nocturnal angina, asthmatic attacks, and duodenal ulceration can occur during these periods of physiologic arousal. Now it is known that the REM-like 90- to 120-min periods ('ultradian rhythm') with concomitant psychophysiologic variability occur during waking life as well. Thus, ultradian rhythm has been shown to be associated with gastric contractility [*Hiatt and Kripke*, 1975], and 'oral' behaviors such as eating, drinking, and smoking [*Friedman and Fisher*, 1967]. If the ultradian rhythm is associated with changes in the mode of thinking, such as the 'primary' process, visual, nonlogical thinking as in dreams, it is possible that, indeed, such altered central nervous system states might provide a particularly favorable opportunity for certain pathogenic psychophysiologic processes to occur.

Rhythmic activities are by no means confined to the ultradian. Most individuals are familiar with their circadian rhythms of sleep-awake cycles. Circadian rhythms are also found in a number of endocrine activities. Memory, drug sensitivity, and conditioned learning, among others, are also influenced by the time of the day. For example, psychotropic drugs were shown to be most effective when administered just before the rest period

[*Stroebel*, 1957]. Slower cycles, such as the menstrual cycle, are of course associated with physiologic changes. Manic-depressive cycles may be seen as an exaggeration of such a slow rhythm. Clearly, there is much need for more investigation in this field.

For psychosomatic medicine, the main implication of recent findings is that biologic rhythmus should be taken into consideration in investigating the pathogenesis and treatment of illnesses.

### Studies on Early Experience and Conditioning

Laboratory behavioral experiments such as conditioning have also produced breakthroughs that have changed views concerning the human organism's learning potential. Autonomic conditioning experiments in the 1960s and 1970s clearly showed that the visceral organs and the circulatory system could 'learn' from experience, and that they could be modified by reward and punishment [*Miller*, 1969].

Studies in early experiences and environments of animals have provided data showing that different early experiences can result in different physiologic and behavioral characteristics. Rats reared in groups were more prone to gastric ulceration after the stress of immobilization, as opposed to rats reared singly [*Ader*, 1965], who were more susceptible to such pathologic conditions as convulsions and mammary tumors. *Leigh and Hofer* [1973] showed that isolation from peers in very early infancy in rats decreased cardiac reactivity to social intrusions but increased behavioral reactivity and fierceness. Whether the effects of early environment, and conditioned responses acquired then, might be incorporated into the constitution of human beings is an important question requiring further studies. For example, would an infant who was fed each time he blanched while crying 'learn' that vasoconstriction was rewarded, and thus develop a tendency to vasoconstrict when encountering frustration?

*Ader and Cohen* [1975] found that immunosuppression could be conditioned in rats by pairing an immunosuppressive agent to a saccharin solution, which was used as a conditioned stimulus. This opens up the possibility that some individuals may learn to respond to certain life events as if they were conditioned stimuli for an organic disease. Would such learning occur more readily in altered states of consciousness?

Medical sociologists have made major contributions to a comprehensive understanding of the behavioral aspects of patienthood. *Parsons* [1964] conceptualized the 'sick role', the social expectations of the ill person. *Mechanic's* [1962] studies concerning how a person behaves in the presence of a symptom, called illness behavior, showed the importance of a number of social factors such as social class and ethnicity. *McWhinney* [1972] proposed a taxonomy of patient behavior, that is, the immediate reasons why a patient-physician contact occurs. His main classifications were (1) limit of tolerance (as of pain or disability); (2) limit of anxiety (for example, anxiety concerning the implications of hemoptysis), and (3) problems of living presenting as a symptom. The third category calls for attention to the possibility that despite the presence of a physical symptom, the patient's immediate need might be in the area of psychosocial problem-solving.

### Newer Developments in Psychiatry

Advances in psychopharmacology have provided effective treatment modalities for a number of psychiatric syndromes seen in medical and psychiatric settings, such as severe anxiety, depression, and psychosis.

Newer treatment modalities, such as biofeedback, using the principles of operant conditioning, potentially provide the means by which individuals may be able to prevent certain disruptive effects of psychologic stress, such as sustained hypertension, or even treat some disorders of the autonomic nervous system and skeletal muscles.

As the main theater of research development in psychiatry shifted from the office to the laboratory, and the black box ceased to be quite so black, with rays of light penetrating into the neurons and the neurotransmitters, the boundary line between psychosomatic investigation and psychiatric investigation proper began to blur. For instance, a theory concerning affective disorders by *Akiskal and McKinney* [1975] posits a model of interaction between the perceptual system related to psychosocial events and the biochemical state of the diencephalon, which may have a genetic vulnerability as a 'given'. The theory of *Prange* et al. [1974] of the affective disorders, with low serotonin level in the brain as a genetic marker, with catecholamine levels correlating with mania or depression, is the classic psychosomatic model along the lines of peptic ulcer [*Weiner* et al., 1957].

Research on possible genetic markers of schizophrenia, such as eye tracking abnormalities [*Holzman* et al., 1974], creatine phosphokinase levels in the serum [*Meltzer*, 1976], abnormalities of neurotransmitters such as dopamine, developmental and family dynamics [*Lidz* et al., 1965], and on

*Table I.* Patient evaluation grid (PEG)

| Dimensions | Contexts | | |
|---|---|---|---|
| | Current (current states) | Recent (recent events and changes) | Background (culture, traits, constitution) |
| Biological | | | |
| Personal | | | |
| Environmental | | | |

the phenomenology and the switching process into psychosis [*Bowers*, 1974], all suggest that the pathogenesis of schizophrenia is also compatible with the psychosomatic model.

## *Development of the Patient Model and the Patient Evaluation Grid*

As a method of applying the modern psychosomatic or systems model in patient care, the patient evaluation grid (PEG) was developed by *Leigh and Reiser* [1980] and *Leigh* et al. [1980].

The PEG uses a three-dimensional approach as in the biopsychosocial model, but proposes that the three dimensions (biological, personal, and environmental) be intersected by three time contexts (current, recent, and background) to form nine squares of investigation for comprehensive understanding of the patient (table I, II).

The PEG has been proposed as an operational method of implementing the 'patient model' – a technique of ensuring that all the relevant personal and environmental information that is necessary in managing the patient is obtained as well as biological information leading to the diagnosis and treatment of the disease. This model does not make any prior assumptions about

*Table II.* Patient evaluation grid

| Dimensions | Contexts | | |
|---|---|---|---|
| | Current (current states) | Recent (recent events and changes) | Background (culture, traits, constitution) |
| Biological | symptoms physical examination vital signs status of related organs medications disease | age recent bodily changes injuries, operations disease drugs | heredity early nutrition constitution predisposition early disease |
| Personal | chief complaint mental status expectations about illness and treatment | recent illness, occurrence of symptoms personality change mood, thinking, behavior adaptation – defenses | developmental factors early experience personality type attitude to illness |
| Environmental | immediate physical and interpersonal environment supportive figure, next of kin effect of help-seeking | recent physical and interpersonal environment life changes family, work, others contact with ill persons contact with doctor or hospital | early physical environment cultural and family environment early relations cultural sick role expectation |

psychosocial factors that may enter into the pathogenesis of disease, but rather facilitates research into the relationships by systematically cataloging such possible factors in the same table that catalogs biological data concerning disease.

It may be noted that all the areas of investigation that led to the development of the modern concept of psychosomatic medicine fit into one or more spaces in the PEG (table III). The PEG also shows that each of the investigative areas must be considered in relationship to other areas of investigation and data derived from them if the patient is to be understood comprehensively.

The practical implication of this model is that a comprehensive evaluation will be performed with each patient in order to complete the PEG, and

*Table III.* Areas of psychosomatic investigation in the PEG

| Dimensions | Contexts | | |
|---|---|---|---|
| | Current (current states) | Recent (recent events and changes) | Background (culture, traits, constitution) |
| Biological | biologic rhythms status of CNS/ANS neurotransmitters hormonal status | immunologic, endocrine, ANS changes related to anxiety, depression, environmental stress drugs biologic rhythms | constitution heredity (e.g. 'serum pepsinogen level') |
| Personal | mental status status of defenses presence of anxiety, depression or psychosis | development of anxiety, depressive mood, changes in behavior changes in coping ability illness behavior | personality pattern (e.g. type A) conflicts (e.g. over dependency) habitual defenses (e.g. denial) |
| Environmental | supportive figures family, friends, work residence environmental state | environmental change (e.g. crowding, life changes, etc.) | sick role expectations cultural and early family influence (e.g. learning to vasoconstrict) |

that possible relationships among factors in different dimensions and contexts may become evident by this single display. Further, by considering factors and problems in the time contexts of current, recent, and background, the urgency of intervention and the ease of treatment becomes clear. Current context factors require immediate attention, recent context factors might have precipitated the current problems, and the background context factors must be considered in the management of the patient (e.g. personality style, predisposition to disease) but are relatively resistant to change.

The PEG ultimately leads to a three-dimensional diagnosis and management plan (which is, in turn, short- and long-term), which may be displayed in the PEG management form (table IV).

The PEG and the recent developments in psychosomatic medicine leading up to this model demonstrate the relationship between the mind

*Table IV.* Patient evaluation grid: management form

| Dimensions | Diagnosis | Therapy plans | |
|---|---|---|---|
| | | short term | long term |
| Biological | | | |
| Personal | | | |
| Environmental | | | |

and the body – these are aspects of the individual's organization and function. The mental status in the personal dimension is the status of the *functioning* brain (or malfunctioning due to chemical toxins). In treating moderate agitation, both drugs and skillful talking can help, and either will result in changes in all biological, personal and environmental dimensions. The PEG also shows *levels* of organization – the aggregation of biological components make up the person (as an entity), who is in interaction with the environment within the ecosystem. Mind and body may be seen to be labels given to different functions of the same organism – the information processing and matter-energy processing functions [*Miller, 1978*].

In a computer, weak electric current or damaged transistor will result in faulty information processing (as in organic brain syndrome) and certain kinds of information or information overload may cause short circuiting or overheating of components (as in stress-related diseases).

### Consultation-Liaison Psychiatry

As awareness of the importance of the psychologic factors in the course of medical illness increased, and as more and more psychiatric units were set up in general hospitals, psychiatrists were called upon more and more frequently for expert advice on medical patients who had concomitant psychiatric problems or whose medical illnesses were thought to be related to emotional stress. That this activity required experience and skills different from those usually expected of a psychiatrist was recognized during a time when psychiatry in general was drifting farther and farther away from other medical and surgical specialties and developing its own jargon and concepts not easily understood by those outside the profession. Thus, the need for careful observation rather than inspired guessing, for jargon-free communication, and for flexibility in the choice of therapy in general hospital psychiatry was acknowledged as early as 1929 [*Henry*, 1929].

In the 1930s, a number of psychiatric consultation-liaison services appeared in general hospitals [for a comprehensive review of the history of liaison programs in the US, see *Greenhill*, 1977]. During the early stages of development the dominant theoretical framework in which the liaison psychiatrist functioned was the linear approach of 'psychogenesis' of psychosomatic disorders. Although this approach provided a conceptual framework that inspired confidence, it also gave rise to the unfortunate stereotype of the psychosomaticist who would try to find 'the unconscious cause' of the medical illness. The idea of psychogenesis in illness also tended to serve the dualism of some nonpsychiatric physicians, who would 'unload' a complex and difficult patient on the psychiatrist once a disease was suspected of being 'psychosomatic'.

## Systems Approach in Consultation-Liaison Psychiatry

As *Lipowski* [1974] pointed out, the essence of consultation-liaison psychiatry today is a comprehensive approach to the patient, in his biologic, psychologic, and social dimensions. This approach is obviously inimical to simple reductionistic ones, whether to unconscious conflicts or twisted molecules. Later developments in psychosomatic medicine along the experimental line mentioned above have reaffirmed the holistic principle, and the modern liaison psychiatrist is a flexible, broadly based physician committed to this approach.

Clinical application of the research findings in psychosomatic medicine in the treatment and evaluation of medical patients is, then, nothing but the practice of good psychiatric principles. Psychosomatic medicine and consultation-liaison psychiatry now ceases to be a separate set of assumptions concerning a limited number of illnesses, but rather an attitude on the part of the consultant psychiatrist. This attitude involves acceptance of all the complex aspects of an individual patient, the biologic, psychologic, and social, as well as their interactions. In the liaison role, the psychiatrist interprets and mediates among all the systems (such as other hospital services, patients, staff, and so forth) involved in the health care delivery system [*Lipowski*, 1974]. For example, he may interpret the patient's behavioral characteristics to the medical staff, and mediate misunderstandings and differences between the patient and staff as well as within the medical staff, using his expertise in the assessment of human behavior.

An understanding of the sociology of the hospital and the influence of the milieu on the patient is essential for liaison work. Attitudes toward the sick role on the part of the doctor and the patient can result in severe misunderstandings and disagreements. For example, a patient whose life style is characterized by the need to control his own environment may have major difficulties in complying with the physicians' orders in the hospital, thereby evoking an angry reaction in the doctor, who may feel the patient is being personally antagonistic. The phychiatrist's interpretation for the primary physician of the patient's personality can help put his behavior in perspective, minimize personal antagonisms, and work out a rational management plan with maximal allowance for the patient's adaptive defensive maneuvers.

Liaison work invariably includes educational activity, not only in specific areas such as the use of psychotropic medications or an approach to patients tailor-made to their personalities, but also in informing the medical staff of the complex interaction of biologic, social, and psychologic factors in the pathogenesis and course of illness and steering them away from a Cartesian dualism of mind and body, perhaps through the use of the PEG.

### Consultation-Liaison Research

As more psychiatrists undertook work in consultation-liaison settings in the general hospital, it became clear that there were certain areas of investigation optimally suited for the liaison psychiatrist. These areas include the psychologic aspects of medical procedures, such as open heart surgery, organ transplantations, and the psychosocial aspects of the hospital environment. How such variables as psychologic defenses influence a medical course is another area of concern. For example, *Hackett* et al. [1968] found that patients who were able to use the mechanism of denial effectively – and this was based simply on whether the patient admitted to feeling or having felt any apprehension or emotional upset in the hospital – had a better prognosis while in the coronary care unit with a myocardial infarction than those who did not deny anxiety. This is a good example of the need for special training for consultation-liaison psychiatrists because the approach to patients who use massive denial in an acute medical setting may be very different from the approach to those in long-term intensive psychotherapy. Clearly, denial in some acute medical settings and situations is advantageous to the patient in terms of the medical course and should be supported rather than 'chipped away'.

*Leigh* et al. [1972] found that subtle changes in the general feeling tones of patients occurred when the coronary care unit of a general hospital changed from a noisy, open, four-bed room to closed, quiet cubicles. In the open, noisy unit patients tended to feel more mutilation and shame anxiety as measured by the Gottschalk-Gleser verbal sample technique, whereas patients in the closed unit felt more separation anxiety. Patients in the closed unit tended to deny and displace their hostile feelings, whereas patients in the open unit were able to express hostile feelings more directly. Of course, the amount of interaction with the staff was greater in the open unit. In addition, they found that regardless of the unit patients who had high separation anxiety, high hostility directed inward (which might be similar to depressive states) and low levels of overt hostility had a significantly greater risk of developing cardiac arrhythmias while in the coronary care unit. Studies such as these point to the need for studies designed to elucidate the interaction between the hospital environment, both physical and psychological, the medical course of the patient, and the personality characteristics of the patient. It may thus be possible to effect optimal treatment of the patient taking into account his personality and his optimal environment.

Increasing numbers of psychiatrists are called on to render opinions concerning issues which fall into the domain of medical ethics and the law. These issues, familiar in the general hospital, include whether patients should be preferentially given or denied the opportunity for an organ transplant because of the personality characteristic, when a patient should be allowed to choose certain death rather than receive treatment, and when a patient is competent to sign out against medical advice or participate in an experiment that might be risky. In regard to some of these issues, we, the liaison psychiatrists, are able to contribute expertise; to others, we are not.

*Future Role of the General Psychiatrist*

We mentioned earlier that in terms of research the distinction between psychosomatic research and psychiatric research has become blurred. We might now say that the boundary line between consultation-liaison psychiatry and general psychiatry is also beginning to blur. What, then, is the appropriate role of the general psychiatrist of the future?

The answer to this question may lie in the recognition that there is a need for physicians who will bridge the gap between the medical and physical sciences on one hand, and the behavioral, social sciences on the other. It takes a doctor to be able to talk to doctors and to teach doctors, it takes a behavioral scientist to grasp the complexities of the social organization of the hospital, the personality of the patient, and the interactions between the psychosocial and medical factors. This is an important role, as neglect of the psychosocial dimension often results in ineffective or shortsighted medical treatment, such as simply treating the vital signs in a patient with an overdose with suicidal intent and then discharging him without follow-up, or on the other extreme, treating a patient with depression associated with the carcinoma of the tail of the pancreas with psychotherapy alone.

This role as a bridge between medicine and behavioral science, and interpreter of both [Reiser, 1973], may be the primary role of the future general psychiatrist. It is clearly the role of the liaison psychiatrist at present. In addition to this primary role, he may develop a secondary, specialized area, such as neuropsychiatry or depth psychotherapy. The liaison psychiatrist also functions as a member of a team of professionals consisting of the nurses, social workers, occupational therapists, and so forth. He works closely with the liaison-nurse specialist who, in the expanded role of nursing, collaborates with and complements the psychiatrist in working with the patient, the nurses, and the liaison team.

*Conclusion*

The modern concept of psychosomatic medicine is, therefore, not of a subspecialty of either medicine or psychiatry that treats defined psychosomatic illnesses, but rather of an attitude that espouses a comprehensive medical practice, utilizing up-to-date psychiatric and neurobiologic knowledge and concepts as well as principles and information gained from the social and behavioral sciences. 'Behavioral medicine', might be useful to denote this modern concept. It has the advantage of eliminating the implied dualism in 'psychosomatic' medicine.

The major theater for the practice of this comprehensive attitude is the general hospital, and those of us who are involved in the practice and teaching of such approaches in the general hospital are practicing psychosomatic medicine. This is, however, only one theater of such a practice; wherever we treat our patients with psychotropic medications, while trying to understand the patient psychologically and his environment through study of family interactions, we are in fact practicing what is the essence of psychosomatic medicine: the integration of the biologic and behavioral sciences.

## References

Ader, R.: Effects of early experience and differential housing on behavior and susceptibility to gastric erosions in the rat. J. comp. Physiol. Psychol. *60:* 223–238 (1965).

Ader, R.; Cohen, N.: Behaviorally conditioned immunosuppression. Psychosom. Med. *37:* 333–340 (1975).

Akiskal, H.S.; McKinney, W.T.: Overview of recent research in depression. Archs gen. Psychiat. *32:* 285–305 (1975).

Alexander, F.: Psychosomatic medicine (Norton, New York 1950).

Bartrop, R.W.; Lazarus, L.; Luckhurst, E.; et al.: Depressed lymphocyte function after bereavement. Lancet *i:* 834–836 (1977).

Bowers, M.B.: Retreat from sanity (Human Sciences Press, New York 1974).

Breuer, J.; Freud, S.: Studies on hysteria; in Strachey, The standard edition of complete psychological works of Sigmund Freud, vol. 11 (Hogarth Press, London 1955).

Bruhn, J.G.; Chandler, B.; Wolf, S.: A psychological study of survivors and non survivors of myocardial infarction. Psychosom. Med. *31:* 8–19 (1969).

Dunbar, F.: Emotions and bodily changes (Columbia University Press, New York 1954).

Engel, G.L.; Schmale, A.R.: Psychoanalytic theory of somatic disorder conversion, specificity, and the disease onset situation. J. Am. psychoanal. Ass. *15:* 344–365 (1967).

Friedman, M.; Rosenman, R.H.: Association of specific overt behavior pattern with blood and cardiovascular findings. J. Am. med. Ass. *96:* 1286–1296 (1959).

Friedman, M.; Rosenman, R.H.: Type A behavior and your heart (Knopf, New York 1974).

Friedman, S.; Fisher, C.: On the presence of a rhythmic diurnal, oral instinctual drive cycle in man: a preliminary report. J. Am. psychoanal. Ass. *15:* 317–345 (1967).

Hackett, T.R.; Cassem, N.Y.; Wishnie, H.A.: The coronary care unit. An appraisal of its psychologic hazards. New Engl. J. Med. *279:* 1365–1370 (1968).

Henry, G.W.: Some modern aspects of psychiatry in general hospital practice. Am. J. Psychiat. *86:* 481–499 (1929).

Henry, J.P.; Stephens, P.M.; Axelrod, J.; Mueller, R.A.: Effect of psychosocial stimulation on the enzymes involved in the biosynthesis and metabolism of noradrenaline and adrenaline. Psychosom. Med. *33:* 227–237 (1971).

Henry, J.; Stephens, P.M.; Watson, F.M.: Force breeding, social disorder and mammary tumor formation in CBA/USC mouse colonies. A pilot study. Psychosom. Med. *37:* 227–283 (1975).

Hiatt, J.E.; Kripke, D.F.: Ultradian rhythms in waking gastric activity. Psychosom. Med. *37:* 320–332 (1975).

Holmes, T.; Rahe, R.H.: The social readjustment rating scale. J. psychosom. Res. *11:* 213 (1968).

Holzman, P.S.; Proctor, L.R.; Levy, D.L.: et al.: Eye tracking dysfunctions in schizophrenic patients and their relatives. Archs gen. Psychiat. *133:* 192–197 (1974).

Jenkins, C.D.: Recent evidence supporting psychologic and social risk factors for coronary disease. Parts 1 and 2. New Engl. J. Med. *294:* 987–994, 1033–1038 (1976).

Kaplan, H.I.: History of psychosomatic medicine; in Kaplan, Freedman, Sadock, Comprehensive textbook of psychiatry/III, vol. 2, pp. 1843–1853 (Williams & Wilkins, Baltimore 1980).

Kennedy, J.A.; Bakst, H.: The influence of emotions on the outcome of cardiac surgery. A predictive study. Bull. N.Y. Acad. Med. *42:* 811–845 (1966).

Kimball, C.P.: Psychological responses to the experience of open heart surgery. J. Psychiat. *126:* 348–359 (1969).

Leigh, H.; Hofer, M.A.: Behavioral and psychologic effects of litter-mate removal on the remaining single pup and mother during the pre-weaning period in rats. Psychosom. Med. *35:* 497–508 (1973).

Leigh, H.; Hofer, M.; Cooper, J.; et al.: A psychological comparison of patients in 'open' and 'closed' coronary care units. J. psychosom. Res. *16:* 449–458 (1972).

Leigh, H.; Feinstein, A.R.; Reiser, M.F.: The patient evaluation grid. A systematic approach to comprehensive care. Gen. Hosp. Psychiat. *2:* 3–9 (1980).

Leigh, H.; Reiser, M.F.: The patient; biological, psychological, and social dimensions of medical practice (Plenum Press, New York 1980).

Lidz, T.; Fleck, S.; Cornelison, A.: Schizophrenia and the family (International University Press, New York 1965).

Lipowski, Z.J.: Review of consultation psychiatry and psychosomatic medicine. III. Theoretical issues. Psychosom. Med. *30:* 395–422 (1968).

Lipowski, Z.J.: Consultation-liaison psychiatry. An overview. Am. J. Psychiat. *131:* 623–630 (1974).

McWhinney, J.R.: Beyond diagnosis – an approach to the integration of behavioral science and clinical medicine. New Engl. J. Med. *287:* 384–387 (1972).

Mechanic, D.: The concept of illness behavior. J. chron. Dis. *15:* 189–194 (1962).

Meltzer, H.Y.: Serum creatin phosphokinase in schizophrenia. Am. J. Psychiat. *133:* 192–197 (1976).

Miller, J.G.: Living systems (McGraw-Hill, New York 1978).

Miller, N.E.: Learning of visceral and glandular responses. Science *163:* 434–445 (1969).

Paclidis, N.; Chirigos, M.: Stress-induced impairment of macrophage tumoricidal function. Psychosom. Med. *42:* 47–54 (1980).

Parsons, T.: Social structure and dynamic process: the case of modern medical practice, in The social system, pp. 428–479 (Free Press Paperback Edition, New York 1964).

Prange, A.; Wilson, I.; Lynn, C.W.; et al.: L-Tryptophan in mania. Contribution to a permissive hypothesis of affective disorders. Archs gen. Psychiat. *30:* 56–62 (1974).

Rees, W.D.; Lutkins, S.G.: Mortality of bereavement. Br. med. J. *iv:* 13–16 (1967).

Reiser, M.F.: Toward an integrated psychoanalytic-physiological theory of psychosomatic disorders; in Lowenstein, Newman, Schur, Psychoanalysis. A general psychology, pp. 570–582 (International University Press, New York 1966).

Reiser, M.F.: Psychiatry in the undergraduate medical curriculum. Am. J. Psychiat. *130:* 565–567 (1973).

Reiser, M.F.: Changing theoretical concepts in psychosomatic medicine; in Reiser, American handbook of psychiatry; 2nd ed., vol. 4, pp. 477–500 (Basic Books, New York 1975).

Rogers, M.P.; Dubey, D.; Reich, P.: The influence of the psyche and the brain on immunity and disease susceptibility. A critical review. Psychosom. Med. *41:* 147–164 (1979).

Schmale, A.H.: Giving up as a final common pathway to changes in health. Adv. psychosom. Med. *8:* 20–40 (1972).

Schur, M.: The ego in anxiety; in Lowenstein, Drives, affects, behavior, vol. 1, pp. 67–103 (International University Press, New York 1953).

Schur, M.: Comments on the metapsychology of somatization. Psychoanal. Study Child. *10:* 110–164 (1955).

Schwartz, G.E.; Weiss, S.: Summary of Proceedings. Yale Conference on Behavioral Medicine. DHEW Pub. No. (NIH) 78-1424 (1978).

Sigerist, H.E.: A history of medicine, vol. 1 (Oxford University Press, New York 1951).

Stein, M.; Schiavi, R.; Camierinio, M.: Influence of brain and behavior in the immune system. Science *191:* 435 (1976).

Stroebel, C.F.: Chronopsychophysiology; in Freedman, Kaplan, Sadock, Comprehensive textbook of psychiatry; 2nd ed., vol. 1, pp. 166–178 (Williams & Wilkins, Baltimore 1957).

Weiner, H.: Psychobiology and human disease (Elsevier North-Holland, New York 1977).

Weiner, H.; Thaler, M.; Reiser, M.F.; Mirsky, I.A.: Etiology of duodenal ulcer. Relation of specific psychological characteristics to rate of gastric secretion (serum pepsinogen). Psychosom. Med. *19:* 1–10 (1957).

Wolf, S.; Wolff, H.G.: Human gastric function; 2nd ed. (Oxford University Press, London 1947).

Zilboorg, G.: A history of medical psychology (Norton, New York 1967).

H. Leigh, MD, Department of Psychiatry, Yale University School of Medicine, 333 Cedar Street, New Haven, CT 06504 (USA)

Adv. psychosom. Med., vol. 11, pp. 23–51 (Karger, Basel 1983)

# Liaison Psychiatry (Liaison Medicine)

*Donald Oken*

Department of Psychiatry, State University of New York,
Upstate Medical Center, Syracuse, N.Y., USA

Liaison psychiatry has assumed a major place within American psychiatry, and medicine as a whole. The past decade, particularly, has witnessed significant growth in the number, size and sophistication of liaison programs. A thorough consideration of the topic is timely.

Indeed, it is necessary, for, remarkably, no focused description of the field exists. Several superb reviews by *Lipowski* [60–64] are most useful. But these fail to concentrate exclusively on *liaison* psychiatry; all deal with *consultation*-liaison psychiatry, blurring the distinction between the two. The same problem besets *Greenhill's* [37] excellent historical overview. It is easy to see how this has occurred. There are real overlaps between these activities, which have been closely linked over the course of their development. But beyond this, programs which subserve either or both functions typically have been indiscriminately designated as 'consultation-liaison' services. This is often a product of ignorance or confusion, though sometimes it is an attempt to imply the presence of liaison where none actually exists. Whatever its basis, this lack of discrimination undermines clear thinking about what each field involves, to the resultant detriment of patient care. One purpose of this present contribution is to make the distinction absolutely clear.

Articles describing specific liaison activities abound. But these are far too circumscribed to give an overall sense of what the purposes and functions of liaison are, how they are accomplished, how such services are organized or, most basically, what liaison 'is'. The definitional problem is, admittedly, a complex one. We will make a beginning here, but allow a fuller and more detailed definition to emerge from a consideration of the development of the field.

Most succinctly, liaison psychiatry can be characterized as the clinical application of psychosomatic medicine. It, therefore, includes *a range of clinically oriented activities which emphasize the integration of psychological and social with biological factors so as to optimize the care of nonpsychiatric patients.* Operationally, it consists of unique collaborative participation in that care – *liaison* – by those who are expert about these factors and their integration, usually selected *psychiatrists*.

To accomplish this, however, requires activities extending beyond direct patient care. Concomitant efforts to modify the knowledge, attitudes and skills of the physicians (and others) primarily responsible for that care are inevitable. The concern widens yet further to the care they will provide other patients. *Educational activities* necessarily merge imperceptibly with those of immediate service as another aspect of the definition.

### Historical Background[1]

#### Origins

The origins of liaison psychiatry necessarily are linked with the development of psychosomatic medicine, which provides its conceptual base. The first substantial foundations were laid during the intellectual ferment of the 19th century [87]. Not until the present century, however, can psychosomatic medicine truly be said to have begun. The stage was set by the 'psychobiology' of *Adolph Meyer* [57, 58, 65] which profoundly shaped all of American psychiatry. Its holistic orientation presaged the general systems theory base [7] which underlies our current conceptualizations; while its 'life chart' approach provided a dynamic approach for viewing transactions between the person and his[2] environment.

But the major conceptual thrust came from psychoanalysis. 'Psychosomatic medicine . . . was an outgrowth of the enlargement of thought brought about by the Freudian revolution' [21]. This provided not only a key frame of reference, but introduced a systematic search for the specifics

---

[1] This section and the entire chapter approach the topic almost exclusively in terms of developments within the United States. Parochial though this may be, I have insufficient familiarity with events elsewhere to do otherwise. It is my impression, moreover, that it is in this country that liaison psychiatry has flowered most extensively.

[2] Throughout this chapter, male terms are used for brevity, by grammatical convention. It should be understood clearly, however, that they are intended to refer to both sexes.

of mind-body relationships, albeit much of this early work is flawed by an undercurrent of simplistic psychologizing. The watershed occurred in the 1930s with the publication of *Dunbar's* [22] epochal *Emotions and Bodily Changes*, *Alexander's* [1] early work, and the initiation of *Psychosomatic Medicine* as the journal of the newly formed American Psychosomatic Society. Psychosomatic medicine had become launched as a scientific and professional field.

Far less noticed at the time, was the first report of consultation-liaison practice. *Henry's* [44] classic 1929 paper provides insights of astonishing durability based on his work with more than 2,000 general hospital patients. From this experience, he concludes the need for all medical students and interns to have psychiatric education based in general hospitals, that emphasizes those disorders which 'complicate general medical and surgical practice', and the need to have psychiatrists in every general hospital, involved in activities of 'mutual exchange'. These points remain valid to this day. And he has much sound advice along the way for the psychiatrist: to keep communications concise, jargon-free and relevant to practical concerns.

During this same decade, important developments were beginning in American psychiatry, then in its infancy as an academic discipline. Much of the impetus came via the assistance of the Rockefeller Foundation under the visionary leadership of *Alan Gregg*. Defining psychiatry 'in its most inclusive interpretation' [76, p. 78], *Gregg* initiated a broad program which provided funds to establish and strengthen university departments of psychiatry, to develop and support research and teaching, and to provide fellowships for advanced training (a number of which were awarded to future leaders in psychosomatic medicine). One specific purpose was 'to bring psychiatry into close relation with other branches of medicine' [75, p. 170]. Several grants were awarded to establish liaison programs in university hospitals.

Important stimulation for this program had come from *Franklin Ebaugh*, and from his 1932 survey of psychiatric education in the US and Canada which documented its abysmal state and isolation from the mainstream of clinical education. Not surprisingly, then, one of the first Rockefeller grants was made to *Ebaugh* at the University of Colorado: 'to secure the services of a psychiatrist to act as a consultant and teacher in the departments of medicine, surgery, obstetrics and pediatrics for the purpose of demonstrating to the students the applicability and usefulness of psychiatric knowledge and the importance of regarding the patient as possibly an individual with mental maladjustment or disease as well as physical illness' [76, p. 89]. This wording is remarkable. It defined at this earliest stage three core characteristics of liaison psychiatry: its locus in other departments, its concern with 'maladjustment' as well as mental 'disease', and the fusion of education with service. With this grant, the 'Psychiatric Liaison Department' was founded at Colorado General Hospital [10–12] – the first known formal use of this term. Less specific beginnings were made elsewhere [40, 94]. World War II then intervened.

### Events Since World War II

Medical experiences in the war sparked great interest in psychiatry and psychosomatic medicine. Psychiatric casualties often were acute, florid and dramatically responsive to psychotherapeutic intervention. Physiological disturbances were a particularly common manifestation [39]. Returning doctors entered psychiatry in large numbers, many with fervor and optimism about the new psychosomatic medicine.

Psychosomatic enterprises abounded during the postwar decade, with psychoanalysts again at the forefront [20]. *Alexander* [2] led the way to a new approach in which the findings of psychoanalysis were related to those from physiology, neurophysiology, endocrinology and other fields. At least one psychoanalytic institute undertook to train internists and other physicians in psychoanalysis. More eclectic training in 'psychotherapeutic medicine' also was conducted [93]. The ties between psychiatry and medicine were strengthened amid great intellectual excitement.

The bubble then began to burst. The emphasis in this new work remained on psychogenesis, which was linked to patterns of personality and their underlying 'psychodynamic constellations', comprehensible only in complex psychoanalytic terms and relevant to a selected group of so-called psychosomatic diseases. It became apparent that this was both oversimplified and restrictive. And even the identified diseases did not respond readily to psychoanalytic therapies. An entire refashioning of clinical and research strategies was required. The field of psychosomatic medicine became discredited in the eyes of many physicians. It seemed dependent upon an esoteric psychology of limited clinical utility relevant solely to a handful of diseases. Even the latter seemed on the verge of yielding to sophisticated new biological approaches.

The increased use of the term liaison psychiatry begins in this period. As *Lipowski* [60] points out, this was partly an attempt to disavow the unfavorable image that had become associated with 'psychosomatic medicine'. The new label was intended to imply an approach of more practical utility relevant across the full range of medicine. It was meant also to convey that the primary concern was patient care, not mere 'academic' pursuits of theory and research.

Constructive though this intent was, we need not throw out the baby with the bath water. Psychoanalytic principles retain their cogency for psychosomatic theory. They are fully compatible with the biopsychosocial model [32] which provides the contemporary conceptual bedrock for both psychosomatic research and clinical work [33]. Moreover, it was from within psychoanalysis that liaison psychiatry largely developed. Those who not only led the way to a holistic reorientation of psychosomatic theory and research, but pioneered the development of liaison services were, for the most part, psychoanalysts: *Grete Bibring, George Engel, Roy Grinker, M. Ralph Kaufman and Eugene Meyer*, among others.

Further, every one of these carried out their work within the *general hospitals* of academic medical centers (as did *Dunbar*). *Lipowski* [64] has noted that 'consultation-liaison psychiatry has developed as an outgrowth of general hospital psychiatric units'. This may seem obvious: It is in general hospitals where (nonpsychiatric) patients and their physicians are to be found. And it is in the challenge of practical confrontation with their problems, and the rubbing of shoulders among psychiatrists and other physicians that liaison naturally emerges. Less apparent is the extent to which these units have burgeoned. The first enduring general hospital psychiatric unit opened in 1929, and by 1939 there were 153 [64]. Following the war, growth accelerated. Their number swelled to 750 by 1970 [64]; and the most recent data reveal that there were 870 in 1979 [3]. (Further, the latter figures omit veterans hospitals, many of which have psychiatric services.) In-patient units comprise the core of most of these programs, but consultation services almost inevitably have developed alongside, or sometimes represent their primary function. A number have evolved to include true liaison services as well.

A vast increase (exceeding 450% [16]) in the numbers of psychiatrists also contributed to the postwar development. Many received valuable tutelage in psychiatric consultation and, to a lesser extent, liaison work during their residencies [69, 83]. Leadership (and funding!) from the National Institute of Mental Health was a crucial factor in supporting these residencies and, more recently, in promoting education in consultation and liaison psychiatry. (*James Eaton* is due particular credit for leadership of the latter [25].) Now, in the 1980s, substantial numbers of psychiatrists are working in many general hospitals, where their skills and enthusiasm have expanded further.

Meanwhile, American medicine as a whole was experiencing a transformation. There was an explosion of knowledge in the biological sciences, with the introduction of innumerable new highly technical devices, and an accelerating sequestration of physicians into specialties and subspecialties. Mutually reinforcing, each served also to make medical care more impersonal and technicized. Triumph after triumph were scored over acute illnesses, obscuring the mounting problems of chronic illnesses. In the initial glow, psychological and social factors seemed of ever dimmer import, if not entirely dispensable. Psychosomatic medicine, its image already tarnished, received scant attention.

Patients however felt quite otherwise, voicing ever louder complaints which medicine could not ignore about dehumanized, fragmented mechanical care. Some of the response was far from optimal: an attempt to engraft humanism on the prevailing bio-medical model as an antidote for its inherent faults; the rise of cults of 'wholistic medicine'; and the partly rational surge to an overromanticized notion of 'primary care'. However, the problem was not too much science, but inadequate science, as *Romano* [77] wisely pointed out. And there were more thoughtful reactions, among them a resurgence of interest and support for liaison psychiatry.

### The Development of Liaison Models

One would be mistaken, however, to conclude that liaison services became common as a result of the various influences described. These have had a very favorable impact on the availability and quality of psychiatric consultation services. In liaison psychiatry, however, the gains have been more modest, with the greatest progress in education. Its potential for growth is now very real, but only very partly realized. Genuine liaison services remain the exception outside of a modest number of major academic medical centers, in a handful of which these services arose. An examination of these pioneering models will be instructive in further delineating our definition of the field.

The Colorado department [10–12] consisted of one psychiatrist, *Edward G. Billings*, assisted by a social worker and secretary. *Billings'* approach emphasized that the liaison psychiatrist 'constantly has to maintain the clinical perspective of his nonpsychiatric colleagues as well as . . . his own specialty' [10]. This cardinal principle of liaison work was facilitated by his own dual training in internal medicine.

Two of the broad aims of the department also retain much of their general validity:

'(1) To sensitize physicians and students to the opportunities offered them by every patient, no matter what complaint or ailment is present, for the utilization of a "common sense" psychiatric approach for betterment of the patient's condition, and for making the patient better fitted to handle his problems – somatic or personality determined or both.

(2) To establish psychobiology as an integral working part of the professional thinking of physicians and students of all branches of medicine.'

Activities in the in-patient services centered on the response to formal referrals only. (It is difficult to see how this could be otherwise, given the availability of but a single psychiatrist.) The descriptions of these referrals suggest that most patients could be given 'psychiatric' diagnoses, with most of the balance were adjudged free of such and requiring more somatic study. Thus, the interplay among biological, social and psychological factors was not a prominent concern. For these reasons, the department served largely a consultative function, rather than true liaison. But all referrals were accepted. *Billings* here articulates another important principle: any requirement of 'selectivity' of referral undermines the aims and credibility of liaison work. The restrictiveness was further ameliorated by *Billings*' attendance once weekly at regular medical ward rounds, an activity since recognized as among the most valuable of liaison techniques. Additionally, *Billings* himself sometimes conducted 'ward walks', or reviewed nonreferred cases on the wards on in medical clinic (where he frequently spent half-days). These latter activities were designed largely for the education of medical students, as were various lectures and other teaching exercises. An interesting feature was the institution of periodic 'Medical-Sociologic Conferences'.

A major shift occurred with the model developed by *M. Ralph Kaufman* at Mount Sinai Hospital in New York in 1946 [6, 49, 51]. The Colorado design was a product of its base in a College of Medicine and a Meyerian orientation. *Kaufman's* perspectives grew from his psychoanalytic orientation and the psychosomatic movement which it spawned. It also reflected a primary concern with general hospital psychiatry, of which he was one of the chief architects [50]. *Kaufman* saw the new postwar psychiatry as, for the first time, having entered 'into the great stream of American medicine' [49, p. 369]. The psychiatrist's role not only transcended mental illness to encompass 'the individual and the complex psychological and emotional factors which might etiologically and concurrently relate to all forms of illness' but extended to the role of 'integrator and catalyst in the teaching . . . and practice of medicine' [49, p. 370].

*Kaufman* designated liaison psychiatry as 'the most significant division for the role of psychiatrists in a general hospital' [49, p. 370], completely inverting its traditional role as ancillary to in-patient services. Liaison psychiatrists were assigned to each of the hospital specialty services and subdivisions. There, each became 'functionally and operationally a member of the medical team' [6, p. 385]. They participated directly in the ongoing activities of that team, and were free to see and follow any patient, whether there was a request for consultation or not. Their opinions often were communicated informally, in person or in brief notes on the chart, rather than via written consultation forms. With these features, the first genuine liaison service came into being.

*Kaufman* addresses other issues. Although an integral member of the team, a psychiatrist must retain his identity as such. Attempts to 'smuggle himself into medicine under false colors', and demonstrate 'that he too is a top internist or surgeon' [49, p. 373] are doomed to failure and derision. And they detract from his unique contributions as specialist and integrator. His contributions, however, must be of practical utility. A 'basic fact of life . . . is the simple and pragmatic one as to whether he is of value to other . . . staff. The surgeon or internist is not interested . . . (in) the psychiatric diagnostic label or . . . an esoteric evaluation of psychodynamic factors for their own sake' but 'in a colleague's help to understand and be of practical assistance in the total evaluation and . . . treatment of any given patient' [49, p. 373].

Some of the characteristics of this program reflect the particular nature of Mt. Sinai: a community hospital while also an academic center, in a locale with unusual resources. *Kaufman* could draw upon a large number of senior psychiatrists willing to serve in a voluntary part-time role, while having fewer full time faculty or residents than a university center. The Michael Reese Hospital in Chicago shared many of these characteristics. Thus, its liaison program borrowed very successfully from *Kaufman's* model, after prior less fruitful endeavors [4]. A later variation with specific applicability to private patient care also was developed there [5]. *Greenhill* [37] points out that the Mt. Sinai model involves low cost and other features which may have applicability to many community hospitals.

The program developed by *George Engel* at Rochester [28, 29, 34, 82] is different in several respects. Drawing from his own background in Internal Medicine and his early collaboration with *Romano* [78], *Engel* uniquely emphasizes the *medical component*. His logic is at least twofold. A foundation in psychiatry is incompletely relevant because it fails to provide sufficient familiarity with patients with somatic illness or with the subtleties of the

medical care system. And psychiatrists who enter that turf often are perceived as an alien discipline, not without some reason. Thus, the Rochester
faculty have been Board-qualified in Internal Medicine (although some are
certified in Medicine, others in Psychiatry) and all hold faculty appoint-
ments in both departments [82].

*Engel* refers to his unit as a 'medical-psychiatric liaison group', or sometimes uses the neutral term 'liaison group'. (Some other programs have
adopted his term, or the shorter 'medical liaison'. The latter also has been
used to refer to a specific liaison actively restricted to a locus in internal
medicine, while other parallel activities are labeled 'surgery liaison', etc.)
Actually, his use of the word, medical, has a dual meaning, referring not
only to specific links with that specialty but to the relationship to the profession generally. The broader relationship to all of medicine is the more important. Liaison teachers may come from any clinical specialty, provided they
have the requisite behavioral science foundation and a liaison orientation.

These provisos are crucial. *Engel* [27] emphasizes the critical distinction
between liaison and 'humanistic medicine'. Liaison work rests neither on
mere good wishes nor hoped-for good public relations, but on providing
more effective patient care by the application of scientific knowledge – what
*Romano* [77] has denoted as 'the *scientific* (my emphasis) humanization of
biology'. The dangers of confusing the two have special meaning today,
when increasing numbers of lay writings and professional publications expound on what they term holistic (or wholistic) medicine. Typically, this is
either a bizarre mixture of naive naturalism and mysticism or emphasizes
the addition of religion to the old reductionist biomedical framework.
Neither represents the psychosomatic approach.

*Engel* and his coworkers have made signal contributions to all aspects
of psychosomatic medicine [81]. These have drawn substantially from psychoanalysis, as did *Kaufman's* work; and there are many similarities between
the two in their conceptual approach to the processes of illness and the clinical work of liaison physicians. However, the Rochester program is more like
that in Colorado in placing a primary emphasis on education rather than
service, perhaps reflecting their common base in colleges of medicine. Others
have emphasized education as a central feature of liaison [52, 68, 89].

But the Rochester program is unique in the extent of this and in its
focus on the medical student, for whom a thorough program was developed.
*Engel's* [26] second year course in psychiatry examines the adaptational processes operating in health and disease from a broad psychosomatic and
developmental framework which stresses the commonalities among 'psy-

chiatric' and 'medical-surgical' disorders. Liaison faculty are involved also in other coursework in both medicine and psychiatry. But a separate 'liaison teaching' program is added as well. The cornerstone are the techniques of interviewing and clinical observation [28, 30, 35]. Basic instruction in these areas is followed by applied activities organic to the regular, required clinical clerkship and externship assignments in medicine. Clinical data are used to demonstrate the presence and interaction among biological, psychological and social factors in the individual patient. A further innovative feature is the use of qualified liaison faculty to serve in regular turn in the traditional role of attending physicians: conducting teaching 'rounds', etc. as faculty internists in the medical wards and clinics.

A second educational focus is a liaison fellowship, another innovative component. The background of fellows is that of any clinical specialty. The goal is to 'broaden (their) general medical background . . . while increasing (their) specific psychological perceptivity and skills' [82]. This program has been an unqualified success. Most of its graduates have gone on to senior faculty or other leadership positions. Many have continued to concentrate specifically in liaison and other psychosomatic work, while others have played an influential role in demonstrating the sophisticated application of the biopsychosocial model to clinical practice within their primary specialties. At least one major liaison service was developed on the Rochester model by a former fellow and faculty member [74].

### Characteristic Features

Earlier, we identified liaison as a range of clinically oriented service and educational activities emphasizing an integrated biopsychosocial approach to patient care carried out by experts working in a unique collaborative role in the medical setting. We can now expand this by specifying the characteristic features of that role and its responsibilities.

*Continuity of presence over time* is a central feature. Liaison activity is ongoing, not episodic. A collaborative role is carved out only as availability and performance are demonstrated over a period of time. Any new team member must earn acceptance and trust. But a variety of specific anxieties, distortions and resistances envelop the liaison role. To all those which inhere to psychiatrists and psychological phenomena, are added fears that the liaison physician will expose other team members as inadequate healers, or capture the control or affections of the patient [4, 15, 37, 72]. Open expressions of suspicion and anxiety, not difficult to manage, are supplemented by subtle patterns of resistance, among them complex avoidance mechanisms, inappropriate and undermined referrals, under- and over-referral, and the setting of traps to seduce erroneous overpsychologizing which is then exposed [4, 60].

The establishment of liaison is a phasic process which unfolds gradually, as described by *Beigler* et al. [4]. *Greenhill* [37] refers to the initial stage as one of 'indoctrination and infiltration'. Knowledge of these processes, along with tact and skill are helpful, but can only exert their effects over time. Someone new, no matter how expert, cannot step into the shoes of a successful predecessor, although his path may be smoothed and the time shortened. Even when accepted, the effectiveness of a liaison physician depends upon his meaningful familiarity with the subtle characteristics of the other team members, of their current group interaction, and of the culture of the particular setting.

Resting on that ongoing relationship as well as maintaining it, the liaison role is *organic to the clinical team*. Liaison succeeds only to the degree that this integration takes place. To the extent that the liaison physician is regarded as an outsider, no matter how expert and helpful, his function is impeded. He must be a full member of that team. Optimum body survival requires that heart, lungs, kidneys, liver, etc., all be present and functionally interactive. An artificial kidney – or an outside consultant – may be of immense value in emergencies or to buy time; but it is no full substitute. Nor are the individual team members of a team any more interchangeable than are organs, though their functions may overlap. The role of each member is defined both by his functions and by the characteristics of the person fulfilling them, including his primary specialty identity. A psychiatrist is a psychiatrist, an internist an internist, and so forth. Each performs differently. Efforts to blur these differences in the service of pseudo-equality or of attempting to pander acceptance only undermines genuine integration.

Psychiatrists, by virtue of interest and training, have represented the vast preponderance of liaison physicians. There is every reason to believe this will continue. *Engel* is quite correct in emphasizing that nonpsychiatrists can be equally effective (likely more so as teachers) if they acquire the necessary psychosocial knowledge and skills. But it is the rare and unusually gifted internist (or other specialist) who can devote the interest, time and effort to do so. These areas, however, are the meat of the psychiatrist. So is a familiarity with the nuances and aberrations of behavior, and a facility with relevant therapeutic interventions. Thus the designation, liaison *psychiatry* seems most generally applicable, although not without its dangers.

One such is the assumption that being a psychiatrist is sufficient. Despite pious proclamations to the contrary, only a minority of psychiatrists hold to a comprehensive biopsychosocial conceptual framework [31]. Even this framework is not sufficient. The liaison psychiatrist must have a comfortable familiarity with work in the (nonpsychiatric) medical setting. Becoming an effective team member in that setting requires a relaxed, knowledgeable acceptance of its values, organization, procedures, argot and the like. This takes effort and interest, as well as time. This is one reason why internists or other 'nonalien' specialists may have it easier at first. But it is no assurance. *Engel* reports the telling anecdote of an internist, working in the first days of a liaison fellowship on the very same medical unit he had just 'left', being addressed by his internist colleagues as 'the psychiatrist' [34]! Among psychiatrists, those who prove most successful often have had a period of medical residency in the course of their training. This experience also is helpful in engendering an honest respect for the expertise of other physicians, and for the personal and professional demands of medical practice. Arrogance is at least as destructive as ignorance to successful performance as a liaison psychiatrist.

### Consultation versus Liaison

Contrasts between the consultation and liaison roles further highlight the definition. *Hackett's* [40] vivid simile captures the difference: 'A consultation service is a rescue squad. . . . Like a volunteer fire fighter, a consultant puts out the blaze and then returns home.' Liaison, however, also includes 'setting up fire prevention programs (and) educating the citizenry about fireproofing'. To extend his analogy, the liaison psychiatrist takes responsibility also for spotting potential 'inflammables', and raising their flash points. Even when one consultant serves for an enduring period, thereby becoming highly valued, his episodic presence precludes carrying out these broader functions.

Both the scope and focus of the two are different. The concern of the liaison psychiatrist is with the operation of psychological and social factors in *every* illness. This strikes to the very core of the definition of liaison work. The fundamental premise of the psychosomatic concept which underlies both its clinical and educational responsibilities is that an understanding of illness – all illness – requires a synthesis of biological, psychological and social factors. The liaison physician's perennial presence and *free access to all patients* in the medical setting enable him to identify the operation of psychosocial issues even in patients in whom these are inapparent, have no seeming consequence for the current episode of illness, or are not immediately troublesome.

The consultant, in contrast, is called in to deal with overt aberrant behavior and to identify and treat *psychiatric* disorders, including the clarification as to whether physical symptoms 'arise from' a psychiatric condition, especially in gray areas such as the somatoform disorders. To the extent that the liaison psychiatrist functions also as a consultant, he too is called to deal with these problems. In doing so, however, he attempts not only to respond to the formal needs of consultation, but to illustrate how these 'psychiatric' problems are best understood as an aspect of the psychosomatic approach to all illness.

### Models of Consultation

Psychiatric consultation, even within its narrower role, has undergone a progressive evolution to a more comprehensive set of functions which has paralleled and drawn upon the concomitant development of liaison psychiatry. Three models of consultation have been described, which represent progressive levels of sophistication and complexity [48]. The *patient-oriented approach* is the traditional, delimited clinical consultation. This retains some utility, especially when acute behavioral aberrations occur. But its restricted focus makes it unable to take account of broader influences on the patient which may be crucial. Unhappily, reliance upon this alone remains common, especially outside the teaching hospital.

The '*consultee-oriented approach*', defined by *Schiff and Pilot* [80] is one variant of what *Caplan* [17] has termed 'client-centered case consultation' in the wider area of mental health consultation. Its scrutiny is directed to the referring physician's overt and covert reasons for consultation, and the nature of his difficulties in understanding or managing the patient. Concern centers on the doctor-patient relationship. *Bibring* [8, 9] and *Kahana and Bibring* [47] provided a sophisticated model based on psychoanalytic insights that spans the two approaches. They clarify the ways in which exaggerated behavioral patterns emerge in the clinical situation as understandable manifestations of basic personality processes; they indicate how these provoke reactions in the hospital staff; and they proceed to show how insights into these patterns can be specifically utilized in management to alleviate the problems.

The '*situation-oriented approach*' described by *Greenberg* [36] applies social psychiatry to the medical setting. *Meyer and Mendelson* [71] have used this to provide a perceptive description of the transactional processes which occur among the staff in the hospital ward milieu which serve both a stimulus for, and product of, patient behavior. They indicate how the liaison psychiatrist can constructively modify these group processes. This perspective has been expanded by others to take note of the influence of role stereotypes which reflect our larger culture, and of their variants within specific medical settings [14, 48].

In actual clinical practice, the distinctions among these approaches are blurred. They are not mutually exclusive, as *Lipowski* [60] has emphasized. The skillful consultant uses variations of all three, selecting whichever can be applied most usefully in a given situation, often shifting from one to another in different phases of the same consultation. But their delineation serves more than heuristic clarification. It helps sharpen the difference between consultation and liaison. The consultant has serious inherent limitations in his capacity to pursue the latter two approaches fully, especially the third. He lacks a reservoir of complete information about the physician, team and milieu. More critically, he lacks the degree of relationship to the others on the team upon which a modification of their insight and behavior rests. The liaison psychiatrist is a better consultant than the consultant. He also does more consultation. Published data reveal that the proportion of general hospital patients for whom formal psychiatric consultation is requested range from 2 to 13% [61, 79, 90]. Yet it is widely agreed that the prevalence of psychiatric disorders in medical populations is much higher, ranging from 15 to 73% [19, 37]. Thus, *Kligerman and McKegney* [55] report figures from two Yale-affiliated hospitals as 3 and 8% consultations, but 39 and 46% prevalence. Further, comparing the different clinical services of these hospitals, they noted a correlation between the frequency of consultations and the amount of liaison work on a given service. On the medical service, where the liaison effort was greatest, the consultation rate was 68%. Similarly, *Hackett* [40] quotes a figure of 10% for consultations throughout the Massachusetts General Hospital; but on the coronary care unit, where liaison was especially thorough, the figure was 33% [18]. And *Torem* et al. [90] note that the institution of active liaison on a ward led to a tenfold rise in referrals. Such differences swell further with the inclusion of the numerous informal consultations that characterize liaison work.

*Lipowski* [64] is correct in stating that consultation and liaison are 'mutually complementary'. Nevertheless, the two sets of functions can be delineated even when carried out by the same person, as *Beigler* et al. [4] have clarified so well. And the relationship is weighted on one side. Except in very rare instances [45], liaison activities subsume consultation functions, which are thereby enhanced and expanded while reinforcing the practical value of the liaison role. In contrast, consultation activities more often than not occur in the absence of genuine liaison (although they may stimulate sufficient eventual interest to lead to the latter). The truth is that most 'consultation-liaison' services are misleadingly so titled. It became important for the National Institute of Mental Health to include in its funding criteria [24] the revealing question: 'Is this truly a liaison service or simply a consultation service?'

### Liaison Activities

#### Clinical Services

Clinical activities have come a long way from the time when the psychiatrist's chief task in the general hospital was to identify psychotics and arrange their commitment. Nearly the full range of diagnostic and therapeutic psychiatric activities are now undertaken. In his consultant role, he is asked to see patients with all categories of psychiatric disturbance [85]. These may represent a happenstance concomitance with a medical condition, psychiatric manifestations or complications of that condition, or a situation in which the symptoms of a psychiatric disorder are primarily somatic. Depression (either as symptom or diagnosis) and organic brain disorders are the most common reasons for referral, whereas major psychoses are infrequent [61]. In his liaison role, he sees all these patients – many of whom he has identified himself – plus others in whom psychological and social factors play a significant role in any illness within the spectrum of the particular medical setting. Significantly, formal consultation requests are uncommon for such patients [61]. Hence, this issue likely will be ignored in the absence of a liaison service.

The nature of the diagnostic activities is self-evident. But these represent only the preliminary step. The evaluation must be translated into succinct, clear, jargon-free terms, and accompanied by equally lucid recommendations for appropriate management and treatment. The formal consultation ends there. But the liaison psychiatrist spends time explaining, clarifying and expanding these reports, and translating many into activities within the therapeutic domain of the other staff. Ultimately, liaison education should allow them to implement many of these themselves. The current partial reality is that a number of physicians will acquire a progressive willingness and capacity to do some of this in the course of their collaboration with a liaison psychiatrist.

Experience reveals that the psychiatric consultant's advice is not only too infrequently sought, but often ignored [13, 61]. (Whether this is any more true than for other specialties is uncertain. Very likely it reflects the inherent limitation of all consultation.) But the modeling of successful application by the liaison psychiatrist enhances the likelihood that his recommendations will be carried out, especially as he is available to provide supervision and support in the process.

Nevertheless, complex therapeutic situations arise inevitably wherein the psychiatrist himself must take the primary responsibility. Direct services are called for most often in providing psychotherapeutic intervention. The principles and techniques common to all psychotherapy remain applicable. But the exigencies of the illness, which may be acute, and the practical demands of the setting commonly require flexible, short-term active techniques that effect a rapid response. One example is *Weissman and Hackett's* [42, 91] 'therapeutic consultation with non-interpretive intervention'. This focuses on the acute conflict within the patient, and utilizes the consultant's complementary response to the dynamic forces involved, without making the latter explicit. *Greenhill's* [37] somewhat similar 'crisis-oriented' model has a more behavioral emphasis, and focuses primarily on life stresses. Generally, techniques of clarification and suggestion are mainstays. Hypnosis and other special techniques may be of value in carefully selected instances. A thorough current knowledge of psychopharmacology is essential.

Where there are adequate numbers of residents or fellows, usually it is they who respond initially to consultation requests. The liaison psychiatrist then serves as a 'supervisor', and follows-up during rounds or other activities. To preserve the liaison pattern, residents should be paired with a specific liaison physician to provide consultations on his clinical service and participate in liaison activities there. If his assignment is of reasonable duration, the resident can develop important relationships with his peers on that service, and provide valuable supplementary liaison at their level.

### Participation in Organized Medical Activities

'Rounds' conducted by the attending physician are probably the most characteristic organized clinical activity in teaching hospitals. These serve the dual purpose of teaching and enhancing patient care. Experience has demonstrated that the liaison psychiatrist's active participation in these is usually his single most useful pursuit, apart from patient care. Numerous variations have proved useful. He may accompany the attending physician, adding comments and raising questions as appropriate; and he may conduct a 'mini-interview' of a patient in the process. He may take the lead role at times, accompanied by the attending or substituting for him. During the latter part of rounds, one or more patients may be discussed in depth in the ward conference room; and the liaison psychiatrist may take responsibility for this, perhaps interviewing the patient.

The house staff are the chief beneficiaries of this educational service effort. But medical students and others will be affected also, possibly even the attending physician. Wise liaison psychiatrists linger when rounds end. This provides an opportunity to pursue issues in greater depth. And often a resident will bring up a problem he was loath to reveal in the presence of his attending. Carefully setting time aside to be available on the ward for informal consultation on this and other occasions is of great value.

Separate 'liaison rounds' may also be useful, especially if scheduled as a regular 'subspecialty' activity, with house staff presence required by the parent service. Sometimes, special rounds or organized group meetings for nursing staff prove helpful, particularly in special care units [43, 54]. The key point is to adapt the methods to meet the characteristics of the setting and the needs of its staff.

The acclimatization and learning which take place during rounds are mutually reinforcing. The liaison psychiatrist both becomes familiar and familiarizes himself with the characteristics of the staff and unit. If a fellow or resident is working with him, the latter may attend both these and the separate 'work rounds' conducted by the house staff. Involvement in the practical 'nitty-gritty' of the latter offers unique opportunity for further contributions to service and peer learning on both sides.

The liaison psychiatrist's presence at medical (etc.) grand rounds and conferences is useful but less important. It may cement the sense of belonging and mutual familiarization. These may provide restricted opportunities for input regarding psychosocial factors in the clinical problem under discussion, although a judicious, light touch is essential.

### Educational Activities

Effective liaison teaching presupposes some fundamental knowledge of psychological and social processes, of the clinical data relevant to these, and at least the rudiments of the techniques for eliciting the latter. Acquisition of the knowledge base commonly is the task of early coursework, usually under the rubric of 'behavioral science', now taught in almost all US medical colleges. Although these courses have grown in sophistication, all too often there is an overreliance on teachers from nonmedical disciplines with emphasis on somewhat esoteric subject matter, or the teaching of traditional basic psychiatry. The clinical skills are the focus of courses in 'interviewing', 'introduction to clinical medicine', and the like. While also increasing in frequency and relevance, the effectiveness of these tends to be limited by an emphasis on the acquisition of facts ('taking a history') in the biological sphere. Liaison faculty can make a very important contribution by correcting these deficiencies, and playing an active role in teaching the basics of comprehensive medicine which should be the real goal of these exercises.

However, this subject matter is generally considered as part of the basic ('preclinical') medical curriculum rather than falling within liaison per se, as an aspect of the clinical teaching of more advanced students and of house officers (residents). As such, the primary educational objective of liaison is the transmission of knowledge about the practical applications of the biopsychosocial model and of the clinical skills which underlie it. With this in mind, it is evident that the observed behavior of the liaison physician as a model for identification is particularly influential. Whether on rounds or displayed in clinical work, the demonstration of his approach, the data which these reveal, and the way he incorporates these into a comprehensive picture of the sick patient are central to the teaching process. This is one way in which the nonpsychiatrist may have an advantage, as *Engel* [29] emphasizes. It is easier for the fledgling to identify with a physician 'like himself' than it is to integrate the behavior of someone of another specialty. But the liaison psychiatrist, perceived as a member of the medical team, is far superior in this role than the consultant. His availability to answer questions as they arise is a further asset. Indeed, he may stimulate or raise many of these himself.

Specific educational activities divorced from the clinical situation have more limited value for house staff and students. Their concerns are primarily clinical; and rounds are their chief device for learning. Some liaison programs have developed special 'correlation' or 'psychosomatic' conferences. The usual experience is that these soon are poorly attended by medical house staff except where their senior staff provide very strong encouragement, especially by attending themselves [38]. These tend to be more acceptable and valued by medical students or by liaison fellows and psychiatry residents rotating through the liaison service. In some instances, these are jointly chaired by a psychiatrist and internist. Though this may prove successful with talented leadership [23], this dichotomous design is self-defeating in one sense: It inherently undermines the unity of the psychosomatic concept it attempts to foster. Didactic conferences, panels and seminars which address psychosomatic topics have proved valuable for liaison fellows and psychiatric residents. But most residents in other fields avoid these, as do many students unless required to attend. Additional exercises appropriate to the specific needs of medical students may be developed. There is much to *Engel's* [33] point that these should emphasize interview technique, effective behavioral observation and the use of these data in a way that leads to formulation of the ill patient rather than mere diagnostic categorization.

There are numerous descriptions of the specific activities of a variety of liaison services. (Examples may be found in the following writings and in the sources they cite: [37, 53, 59, 60, 73, 88, 95].) Each is slightly different in ways that reflect its particular leadership, history, and setting. But the overall lessons are clear: the most effective activities, in general, are those closest to the clinical situation and to the setting itself.

### Research

Liaison psychiatrists may be involved in research along with their other activities. This can involve any area of psychiatry, but is likely to deal with psychosomatic phenomena and their underlying mechanisms, or relate directly to their liaison work. But essentially all these latter studies have been merely anecdotal and descriptive. Only the barest beginnings of *systematic* research on liaison service or education exist thus far [46].

Evaluation research which demonstrates the tangible benefits which result from liaison services is a critical current need. Liaison psychiatrists have long believed that their patients tend to improve faster, reach higher levels of functioning and have fewer rehospitalizations. But this has been difficult to prove. Recently, an important study has provided the first hard data bearing on this. *Levitan and Kornfeld* [56] studied matched groups of elderly patients hospitalized for fractures of the femur. The care of one group included participation by a liaison psychiatrist. That group had a significantly shorter hospital stay and twice the rate of return to their own homes, rather than to a nursing home, compared with the controls. More research of this type is necessary.

The broader need is for studies which clarify the advantages and disadvantages of different types of programs, and clinical approaches, for different types of patients. We also need more studies of the effectiveness of liaison programs on our 'educational consumers', especially medical students and house staff. These must go beyond cognitive learning to determine how their behavior as physicians is affected, and how lasting this effect is.

## Organization of a Liaison Service

One individual can provide effective liaison in a limited setting, usually a single hospital unit. Often he will be called upon soon to provide some consultation services elsewhere in the hospital. The start may be on an internal medicine or another general clinical service. Or a psychiatrist's particular interest may gravitate him to a special care unit (intensive care, coronary care, renal dialysis, burn treatment, etc.) where the needs of patients and staff can be intense, the welcome warmer, and the possibilities for research more abundant. Despite these advantages, isolated work is difficult to sustain. The lone liaison psychiatrist usually hopes that such 'islands of excellence' will provide so compelling an example that others will be attracted and wider support generated. If matters go well, he and other hospital leaders will recruit and educate others to begin additional liaison efforts.

There is no formula to define how many liaison psychiatrists a hospital should have. Ideally, their number should grow until all clinical specialty services are covered. In reality, it will be determined by economics, the scope of the hospital's educational commitment, the degree of tangible support by department chairmen and hospital administrators, the availability of qualified psychiatrists, and the extent of medical staff acceptance.

At some critical mass, perhaps as few as two, a liaison 'service' (division, section, etc.) is born. The formal establishment of an organizational entity based in defined office space with secretarial support is a critical step in the long-term viability of the service. Organizational status represents a significant factor in the *realpolitik* and hierarchical bureaucracy of the hospital, as well as offering the advantages of better administration. But the benefits go beyond this. It is stressful to be the sole psychiatrist working on another's turf. Self-esteem and professional identity are threatened. Our successes need not blind us to the facts that a fundamental lack of appreciation – if not actual opposition – to the biopsychosocial model is prevalent in medicine; that few physicians find psychological and social concepts acceptable or even congenial; and that psychiatrists continue to be regarded with suspicion [37, 60, 66, 86]. The nonpsychiatrist in the liaison role fares little better, and must face the feeling that he no longer 'belongs' to his own specialty [34].

Organizational structure provides a mechanism wherein supportive interaction among the individuals of the service can counteract isolation and offer a positive, special identity. This atmosphere facilitates constructive self-evaluation, within which the individuals can recognize and correct the counter-transference distortions inherent in liaison work [70]. Members also share information, hospital gossip and 'tricks of the trade', exchange knowledge about the field, and develop educational activities for their intellectual stimulation and professional growth. The organization also is a vehicle for developing educational programs for trainees, and perhaps liaison fellowships.

Multiple reasons, transparent by now, dictate that a liaison service ordinarily will be a component of the psychiatry department. Even if it is dually affiliated, this is where it will be based almost invariably. Active support of the chairman of psychiatry is needed to ensure adequate resources, including the assignment of residents; and it is crucial as a force 'promoting' liaison throughout the power structure of the hospital, and defending it within the department. At least one key member of the liaison staff must be full time to ensure smooth administrative function. Others will have to devote significant time too; liaison cannot function on a 'catch as catch can' basis. In academic settings, several full time faculty will be involved. Each requires office space, secretarial services and, of course, a salary, most of which must come from the psychiatry budget. Typically, the liaison psychiatrist does much more than that work. His interests as a psychiatrist dictate seeing his own patients, and involvement in educational activities, and perhaps research. These help sustain his identity as a psychiatrist, both for himself and in the eyes of his departmental colleagues, 'justifying' departmental support of liaison activities, and reducing his sense of isolation.

Liaison work can be fraught with feelings of being different, alone and apart. The conceptual frame is no more understood and accepted by psychiatrist colleagues than other physicians [31, 67]. Much of the work is done invisibly, away from them and for others. It is, in fact, different from most other special interest areas in psychiatry (and more so for other specialties). Further, the liaison psychiatrist comes as an 'alien' to work alone among a team whose acceptance is hard won, tenuous and rarely complete. It takes a different type of person to maintain a sense of worth and identity under these circumstances – a difference which may add to feelings of separateness. Meticulous attention to organizational arrangements, thus, is vital.

Backing from chairmen of other departments, particularly internal medicine, can be important. At the least, passive acceptance is required. Space within the clinical or office facilities of these departments is rarely necessary, though sometimes convienent (this may assume quite different importance, however, for the nonpsychiatrist liaison physician). Of greater consequence is the formal scheduling of liaison rounds as official activities of the recipient service [38]. Still better, though rare, is the presence at these exercises of the chief and other senior staff. Support for at least part of the liaison salaries can be a godsend, and adds the dividend of transmitting perhaps the most powerful message of the true import accorded an activity.

### Financial Considerations

Economics is always a problem. A pure consultations service may generate sufficient funds from fee-for-service to be self-supporting. But too much of liaison work involves informal and unsolicited consultation, follow up, and educational activities to permit self-sufficiency. Until recently, federal educational grants took up substantial slack for some programs. But these are fast dwindling, and likely soon to disappear (perhaps by the time this chapter appears) in the fiscal climate of the early 1980s. Hard pressed as they are, departments of psychiatry will have to continue to provide the lion's share of funding.

Financial support from the central hospital administration or the dean of the medical college may prove a solution. The basis for this could not be sounder. Liaison services benefit all clinical services and all educational programs, and may contribute to research. Administrators may acknowledge the benefits to patient care, but are likely to view this as a luxury bought at greater cost. Yet actual savings can result from effective liaison, as the aforementioned research of *Levitan and Kornfeld* [56] has demonstrated. With more research of this type, we may be able to convince administrators of the investment worth of 'front end funding' of liaison psychiatry in hard dollars, as well as for quality care and education.

### Organizational Relationships to the Hospital

*Strain* [88] has provided a valuable analysis of the organizational 'anatomy of the modern teaching hospital' and its implications vis-à-vis liaison psychiatry. Clinical departments typically are separate hierarchical 'fiefdoms', loosely linked in an advisory bureaucracy. Senior faculty are selected more for their research and scholarly accomplishments than their expertise – or even interest – in patient care. The technization of contemporary medical care reaches its acme in such tertiary care institutions, resulting in a mechanized environment. House staff and attending physician assignments are rapidly rotated, nurse turnover is high, and patients are transferred frequently from one special care unit to the next. The liaison psychiatrist may be literally the only clinician available longitudinally over the full course of a patient's stay. He may be the only senior physician primarily concerned with patient care and, as such, the only such role model for house staff. Likely also he will be the only one interested in the 'mental life' of the house staff, as well as the patients.

*Strain* [88] emphasizes that the chief of the liaison service may be able to modify this system most fundamentally via his access to the hospital administrative hierarchy. This structure not only controls the freedom of the liaison psychiatrist to work, but determines hospital policies which define the nature of patient care. The procedures and rules through which a hospital is run determine the extent to which a patient will be considered as a person rather than a biomechanical object. The tone thus set becomes a powerful force in inculcating this value in its residents and other staff.

### Other Disciplines

All the preceding discussion has referred to liaison as a *medical* field. This is not unintended. Beyond the fact that liaison professionals are preponderantly physicians, is the sense that this is a field of medical care that must be led by physicians who know and can respond to the needs of other physicians.

There is also the factor of role modeling. It is difficult enough to transmit the biopsychosocial approach to doctors in training by having their respected seniors display its application within the fabric of medical practice. To suggest that it belongs to an outside discipline is to directly contradict its core message that it represents comprehensive *medicine*.

Yet, other disciplines are active, valuable contributors too. What these others do, however, is represent only part functions of the overall field of liaison work, primarily its consultative component. Clinical psychologists are much the largest group. Well-trained psychologists possess excellent diagnostic and psychotherapeutic skills which can be called upon. Those who have had experience in medical settings acquire a sophistication about the processes involved in disease and medical care, which enhances their effectiveness. Those who have grounding in behavioral approaches provide this added treatment dimension, the usefulness of which has quickly been demonstrated and doubtless will grow further [92]. And, of course, a number are superbly fitted to conduct psychosomatic research. Nevertheless, their inappropriateness for assuming the full liaison role deserves emphasis because there has been a disturbing tendency for a few clinical departments – most commonly family medicine departments – to hire psychologists' services and avoid psychiatrists. The motives behind such a decision are complex, but include a basic resistance to genuine liaison. In any event, they get something much less than this.

Nurses also have been active in liaison programs. They have been particularly valuable in working with the medical-surgical nursing staff who are providing care for a difficult patient. Within their own discipline, they can serve effectively in a role which parallels that of the liaison psychiatrist. They also make a useful contribution to the clinical team by clarifying how patient behaviors affect nursing staff and nursing practice, a function for which they are uniquely suited.

A well-developed liaison division typically includes psychologists, a nurse or two, and often a social worker, in addition to its core of psychiatrists. Or members of these disciplines may join liaison activities on a part-time or case-by-case basis. The psychiatrist's regular liaison activities are thus supplemented by diverse skills which can be called into play as dictated by the best interests of his patients, as well as special educational and research needs.

But there is no one ideal staffing pattern or organizational design, just as there is no single model for the scope and nature of liaison activities. All reflect the history, characteristics, and resources of the setting. The key is to adapt to the local circumstances in whatever ways best promulgate the underlying model of comprehensive patient care throughout its clinical and educational programs.

### Coda

As with all of medicine, the ultimate goal of liaison psychiatry is to make itself superfluous. Were all physicians to master the biopsychosocial underpinning of medicine and its practical applications within patient care, the need for our services would disappear. There is scant possibility that such a goal will be reached for a long, long time to come in any hospital, much less universally. We need have no fear of becoming obsolete! Our problems are quite the reverse. At best, we are educators in a field still in its early stage, with much to teach and more to learn about it ourselves. At worst, we remain pleaders, doctor-chasers, and ear-clutchers [88], striving to get some small part of our essential message heard. The road is, in fact, a hard one, with much distance left to travel.

If I have laid stress upon this and the problems inherent in the liaison role, it has been for descriptive completeness. But there is quite another side. Liaison work is vastly satisfying. No other area provides greater intellectual excitement; richer opportunities for delving into fascinating complexity and working towards new insights; or warmer satisfactions in contributing to the well being of those who are ill. Its rewards are unsurpassed. I commend it with enthusiasm.

## References

1    Alexander, F.: The medical value of psychoanalysis (Nortin, New York 1936).
2    Alexander, F.: Psychosomatic medicine (Norton, New York 1950).
3    Bachrach, L.L.: General hospital psychiatry. Overview from a sociological perspective. Am. J. Psychiat. *138:* 879–887 (1981).
4    Beigler, J.S.; Robbins, F.P.; Lane, E.W.; Miller, A.A.; Samelson, C.: Report on liaison psychiatry at Michael Reese hospital, 1950–1958. Archs Neurol. Psychiat. *81:* 733–746 (1959).
5    Beigler, J.S.: Experiences of liaison psychiatry on a private medical service. Psychiat. Med. *3:* 75–79 (1972).
6    Bernstein, S.; Kaufman, M.R.: The psychiatrist in a general hospital. J. Mt Sinai Hosp. *29:* 385–394 (1962).
7    Bertalanffy, L. von: General systems theory (Braziller, New York 1968).
8    Bibring, G.L.: Psychiatry and medical practice in a general hospital. New Engl. J. Med. *254:* 366–372 (1956).
9    Bibring, G.L.: Psychiatric principles in casework. J. Soc. Casework *30:* 230–235 (1949).
10   Billings, E.G.: Teaching psychiatry in the medical school general hospital. J. Am. Med. Ass. *107:* 635–639 (1936).
11   Billings, E.G.: Liaison psychiatry and intern instruction. J. Ass. Am. Med. Coll. *14:* 375–385 (1939).
12   Billings, E.G.: The psychiatric liaison department of the University of Colorado medical school and hospitals. Am. J. Psychiat. *122:* suppl., pp. 28–33 (1966).
13   Billowitz, A.; Friedson, W.: Are psychiatric consultants recommendations followed? Int. J. Psychiat. Med. *9:* 179–189 (1978–1979).
14   Brodsky, C.M.: A social view of the psychiatric consultation. Psychosomatics *8:* 61–68 (1967).
15   Brodsky, C.M.: Decision-making and role shifts as they affect the consultation interface. Archs gen. Psychiat. *23:* 559–565 (1970).
16   Brown, B.S.: The life of psychiatry. Am. J. Psychiat. *133:* 489–495 (1976).
17   Caplan, G.: Types of mental health consultation. Am. J. Orthopsychiat. *33:* 470–481 (1963).
18   Cassem, N.H.; Hackett, T.P.: Psychiatric consultation in a coronary care unit. Ann. intern. Med. *75:* 9–14 (1975).
19   Denney, D.; Quass, R.M.; Rich, D.C.; et al.: Psychiatric patients on medical wards. Archs gen. Psychiat. *14:* 530–535 (1966).

20    Deutsch, F.: The psychosomatic concept in psychoanalysis (International University Press, New York 1953).

21    Dubos, R.: Man, medicine and environment (Praeger, New York 1968).

22    Dunbar, F.: Emotions and bodily changes (Columbia University Press, New York 1935).

23    Early, L.W.; Gregg, L.A.: A long-term experience with joint medical-psychiatric teaching. J. med. Educ. *34:* 972–1030 (1959).

24    Eaton, J.S.; Haas, M.R.; Abraham, A.S.; Revs, V.I.; Goldberg, R.: The development of criteria for evaluating psychiatric education programs. Archs gen. Psychiat. *33:* 439–442 (1976).

25    Eaton, J.S.; Goldberg, R.; Rosinski, E.; Allerton, W.S.: The educational challenge of consultation liaison psychiatry. Am. J. Psychiat. *134:* suppl., pp. 20–23 (1977).

26    Engel, G.L.: Psychological development in health and disease (Saunders, Philadelphia 1962).

27    Engel, G.L.: Humanism and science in medicine; in Brill, Psychiatry in medicine (University of California Press, Berkeley 1962).

28    Engel, G.L.: Medical education and the psychosomatic approach. J. psychosom. Res. *11:* 77–85 (1967).

29    Engel, G.L.: Training in psychosomatic research. Adv. psychosom. Med. *5:* 16–24 (1967).

30    Engel, G.L.: The education of the physician for clinical observation. J. nerv. ment. Dis. *154:* 159–164 (1972).

31    Engel, G.L.: Is psychiatry failing in its responsibility to medicine? Am. J. Psychiat. *128:* 1561–1564 (1972).

32    Engel, G.L.: The need for a new medical model. A challenge for biomedicine. Science *196:* 129–136 (1977).

33    Engel, G.L.: The clinical application of the biopsychosocial model. Am. J. Psychiat. *137:* 535–544 (1980).

34    Engel, G.L.; Greene, W.L.; Reichsman, F.; Schmale, A.; Ashenberg, N.: A graduate and undergraduate teaching program on the psychological aspects of medicine. J. med. Educ. *32:* 859–871 (1957).

35    Engel, G.L.; Morgan, W.L.: Interviewing the patient (Saunders, Philadelphia 1973).

36    Greenberg, I.M.: Approaches to psychiatric consultation in a research hospital setting. Archs gen. Psychiat. *3:* 691–697 (1960).

37    Greenhill, M.H.: The development of liaison programs; in Usdin, Psychiatric medicine, pp. 115–191 (Brunner-Mazel, New York 1977).

38    Greenhill, M.H.; Kilgore, S.R.: Principles of methodology in teaching the psychiatric approach to medical house officers. Psychosom. Med. *12:* 38–48 (1950).

39    Grinker, R.R.: Men under stress (Blakiston, Philadelphia 1945).

40    Hackett, T.P.: Beginnings. Liaison psychiatry in a general hospital; in Hackett, Cassem, Massachusetts General Hospital handbook of general hospital psychiatry, pp. 1–14 (Mosby, St. Louis 1978).

41    Hackett, T.P.; Cassem, N.H.: Massachusetts General Gospital handbook of general hospital psychiatry (Mosby, St. Louis 1978).

42    Hackett, T.P.; Weisman, A.D.: Psychiatric management of operative syndromes. Psychosom. Med. *22:* 267–282, 356–372 (1960).

43   Hay, D.; Oken, D.: The psychological stresses of intensive care unit nursing. Psycho-
     som. Med. *34:* 109–118 (1972).
44   Henry, G.W.: Some modern aspects of psychiatry in general hospital practice. Am.
     J. Psychiat. *9:* 481–489 (1929–1930).
45   Hockaday, W.J.: Experiences of a psychiatrist as a member of a surgical faculty.
     Am. J. Psychiat. *117:* 706–708 (1961).
46   Houpt, J.: Evaluating liaison program effectiveness. The use of unobtrusive mea-
     surement. Int. J. Psychiat. Med. *8:* 361–370 (1977–1978).
47   Kahana, R.J.; Bibring, G.L.: Personality types in medical management; in Zinberg,
     Psychiatry and medical practice in a general hospital (International University Press,
     New York 1964).
48   Karasu, T.B.; Hertzman, M.: Notes on a contextual approach to medical ward
     consultation. The importance of social system mythology. Int. J. Psychiat. Med.
     *5:* 41–49 (1974).
49   Kaufman, M.R.: The role of the psychiatrist in a general hospital. Psychiat. Q. *27:*
     367–381 (1953).
50   Kaufman, M.R.: The psychiatric unit in a general hospital (International University
     Press, New York 1965).
51   Kaufman, M.R.; Margolin, S.G.: Theory and practice of psychosomatic medicine
     in a general hospital. Med. Clins N. Am. *32:* 611 (1948).
52   Kimball, C.P.: Liaison psychiatry: of approaches and ways of thinking and be-
     havior. Med. Clins N. Am. Vol. 2, No. 2, 201–210 (1979).
53   Kimball, C.: Symposium on liaison psychiatry. Med. Clins N. Am. Vol. 2, No. 2 (1979).
54   Klagsbrun, S.C.: Cancer, emotions, and nurses. Am. J. Psychiat. *126:* 1237–1244
     (1970).
55   Kligerman, M.J.; McKegney, P.: Patterns of psychiatric consultation in two
     general hospitals. Psychiat. Med. *2:* 126–132 (1971).
56   Levitan, S.J.; Kornfeld, D.S.: Clinical and cost benefits of liaison psychiatry. Am.
     J. Psychiat. *138:* 790–793 (1981).
57   Lidz, T.: Adolph Meyer and the development of American psychiatry. Am. J.
     Psychiat. *123:* 320–332 (1966).
58   Lief, A.: The commonsense psychiatry of Dr. Adolph Meyer (McGraw-Hill, New
     York 1948).
59   Linn, L.: Frontiers in general hospital psychiatry (International University Press,
     New York 1961).
60   Lipowski, Z.J.: Review of consultation psychiatry and psychosomatic medicine.
     I. General principles. Psychosom. Med. *29:* 153–171 (1967).
61   Lipowski, Z.J.: Review of consultation psychiatry and psychosomatic medicine.
     II. Clinical aspects. Psychosom. Med. *29:* 201–224 (1967).
62   Lipowski, Z.J.: Review of consultation psychiatry and psychosomatic medicine.
     III. Theoretical issues. Psychosom. Med. *30:* 395–422 (1968).
63   Lipowski, Z.J.: Consultation-liaison psychiatry. An overview. Am. J. Psychiat. *131:*
     623–630 (1974).
64   Lipowski, Z.J.: Consultation-liaison psychiatry. Past, present and future; in Pasnau,
     Consultation liaison psychiatry, pp. 1–28 (Grune & Stratton, New York 1975).
65   Lipowski, Z.J.: Holistic-medical foundations of American psychiatry. A bicentennial.
     Am. J. Psychiat. *138:* 888–895 (1981).

66  Lipsett, D.R.: Some problems in the teaching of psychosomatic medicine. Int. J. Psychiat. Med. *6:* 317–329 (1975).

67  McKegney, F.P.: Consultation-liaison teaching of psychosomatic medicine. Opportunities and obstacles. J. nerv. ment. Dis. *154:* 198–205 (1972).

68  McKegney, F.P.: The teaching of psychosomatic medicine. Consultation-liaison psychiatry; in Reiser, American handbook of psychiatry; 2nd ed., vol. IV, pp. 905–922 (Basic Books, New York 1975).

69  Mendel, W.M.: Psychiatric consultation education – 1966. Am. J. Psychiat. *123:* 150–155 (1966).

70  Mendelson, M.; Meyer, E.: Countertransference problems of the liaison psychiatrist. Psychosom. Med. *23:* 115–122 (1961).

71  Meyer, E.; Mendelson, M.: Psychiatric consultations with patients on medical and surgical wards. Patterns and processes. Psychiatry *24:* 197–220 (1961).

72  Oken, D.: The doctor's job revisited. Psychosom. Med. *40:* 449–461 (1978).

73  Pasnau, R.O.: Consultation-liaison psychiatry (Grune & Stratton, New York 1975).

74  Reichsman, F.: Teaching psychosomatic medicine to medical students, residents and postgraduate fellows. Int. J. Psychiat. Med. *6:* 307–316 (1975).

75  Rockefeller Foundation: Annual Report, 1933.

76  Rockefeller Foundation: Annual Report, 1934.

77  Romano, J.: Basic orientation and education of the medical student. J. Am. med. Ass. *143:* 409–412 (1950).

78  Romano, J.; Engel, G.L.: Teaching experiences in general hospitals. Am. J. Orthopsychiat. *17:* 602–604 (1947).

79  Sasser, M.; Kinzie, J.D.: Evaluation of medical-psychiatric consultation. Int. J. Psychiat. Med. *9:* 123–134 (1978–1979).

80  Schiff, S.K.; Pilot, M.L.: An approach to psychiatric consultation in the general hospital. Archs gen. Psychiat. *1:* 349–357 (1959).

81  Schmale, A.H.; Ader, R.: The challenge of the biopsychosocial model. Psychosom. Med. *42:* suppl., pp. 77–230 (1980).

82  Schmale, A.H.; Greene, W.A.; Reichsman, F.; Kehoe, M.; Engel, G.L.: An established program of graduate education in psychosomatic medicine. Adv. psychosom. Med. *4:* 4–13 (1964).

83  Schwab, J.J.: Consultation-liaison training program; in Mendel, Solomon, The psychiatric consultation, pp. 33–40 (Grune & Stratton, New York 1968).

84  Schwab, J.J.: Handbook of psychiatric consultation (Appleton-Century-Crofts, New York 1968).

85  Schwab, J.J.; Clemmons, R.S.: Psychiatric consultations. Archs gen. Psychiat. *14:* 504–508 (1966).

86  Silverman, A.J.: Lacunae of ignorance, foci of understanding. Psychosom. Med. *39:* 213–218 (1977).

87  Stainbrook, E.: Psychosomatic medicine in the nineteenth century. Psychosom. Med. *14:* 211–227 (1952).

88  Strain, J.J.; Grossman, S.: Psychological care of the medically ill. A primer in liaison psychiatry (Appleton-Century-Crofts, New York 1975).

89  Strain, J.J.: Psychological interventions in medical practice (Appleton-Century-Crofts, New York 1978).

90   Torem, M.; Saravay, S.M.; Steinberg, H.: Psychiatric liaison. Benefits of an 'active'
     approach. Psychosomatics *20:* 598–611 (1979).
91   Weisman, A.D.; Hackett, T.P.: Organizational function of a psychiatric consul-
     tation service. Int. Rec. Med. *173:* 306–311 (1960).
92   Williams, R.B.; Gentry, W.D.: Behavioral approaches to medical treatment (Bal-
     linger, Cambridge, Mass. 1977).
93   Witmer, H.L.: Teaching psychotherapeutic medicine (The Commonwealth Fund,
     New York 1947).
94   Zinberg, N.E.: Introduction. The development and operation of a psychiatric ser-
     vice; in Zinberg, Psychiatry and medical practice in a general hospital, pp. 1–14
     (International University Press, New York 1964).
95   Zinberg, N.E.: Psychiatry and medical practice in a general hospital (International
     University Press, New York 1964).

D. Oken, MD, Department of Psychiatry, State University of New York,
Upstate Medical Center, Syracuse, NY 13210 (USA)

Adv. psychosom. Med., vol. 11, pp. 52–61 (Karger, Basel 1983)

# Practical Distinctions between Consultative Psychiatry and Liaison Medicine

*Daniel S.P. Schubert*

Case Western Reserve University School of Medicine and Cleveland Metropolitan General Hospitals, Cleveland, Ohio, USA

## Introduction

This chapter is one of two with the purpose of introducing reports on consultation-liaison activities in various countries in the world. I am discussing the 'practical' distinction between consultative psychiatry and 'liaison medicine'. The latter will be further defined in a subsequent section. The term 'medical liaisonist' has been proposed by *Engel* [1980] and has been also earlier described by *Reichsman* [1974] as well as in other publications. This chapter will focus on *consultative psychiatry* and will contrast it with *liaison medicine*.

Comparison of consultative psychiatry to liaison medicine is not a dialectic process. The ultimate clinical goal of both endeavors is to enhance patient care. A one-sided advocacy of consultative psychiatry would seem not only to ignore facts of the case, but also to be less useful to readers as an introduction to the later chapters in this volume.

## Definitional Differences between the 'Medical Liaisonist' and the Psychiatric Consultant

The editors have given us definitions of the 'medical liaisonist' and psychiatric consultant.[1] The concept of 'medical liaisonist' as has been proposed

---

[1] Editor's note: These heuristic definitions were included in instructions to the authors. Their antithetical *categorical* denotation is merely useful for purposes of illustration. In fact, as Dr. *Schubert* notes, consultation and liaison work exists along a dimension.

by *Engel* [1980] and *Reichsman* [1974]. The 'medical liaisonist' is part of the department, team or unit in which he works other than psychiatry. He also preferably has a background in a nonpsychiatric medical discipline such as internal medicine. If the liaison worker is a psychiatrist, then he must have knowledge and skills of a nonpsychiatric specialty in addition to his psychosocial expertise. The psychiatric consultant, on the other hand, is a psychiatrist who does not become part of a nonpsychiatric department team or unit. His identification remains clear as a psychiatrist. Thus, the 'medical liaisonist' merges into the nonpsychiatric unit while the psychiatric consultant does not become an integral part of the units to which he consults. The consultant psychiatrist must have training as a psychiatrist. The 'medical liaisonist' may be a psychiatrist but has psychosocial expertise and also has expertise in the nonpsychiatric specialty of which he is a part.

Thus, the consulting consultation psychiatrist retains identity as a psychiatrist while the 'medical liaisonist' may have a more blurred double image of psychosocial expert as well as some expertise in a nonpsychiatric field. It would seem likely from these definitions that the consulting psychiatrist would tend to be primarily a member of the Department of Psychiatry and only secondarily, if at all, a member of a nonpsychiatric department.

### Implications of the Definition

The 'medical liaisonist' is directly stated to be a part of the nonpsychiatric unit and therefore full-time in liaison-type activities. The psychiatric consultant, on the other hand, would seem to usually be less than a full-time consultant to a specific unit.

Training is more differentially specified. The consulting psychiatrist is trained as a psychiatrist. The 'medical liaisonist', on the other hand, is a psychosocial expert and does not necessarily have psychiatric training. In addition, there is at least some expertise in the nonpsychiatric area for the medical liaisonist. Such nonpsychiatric expertise could reflect a varied types of nonpsychiatric training from full board certification to only 1 extra year of nonpsychiatric residency. There are many practicing psychiatric consultants. On the other hand, the 'medical liaisonists' are relatively unusual. If the definition had required a certain minimum of psychosocial knowledge such as a year of training, or a minimum of nonpsychiatric knowledge, again with a specified amount of training, the number of practicing 'medical liaisonists' would probably shrink further. On the other hand, there are many consultative psychiatrists who do also have partial to full training in other medical specialties such as internal medicine, obstetrics, and pediatrics.

### Advantages of Being a 'Medical Liaisonist'

*Engel* [1980] and *Reichsman* [1974] propose that one main advantage of the 'medical liaisonist' is that the nonpsychiatric physician or medical student may find that the 'medical liaisonist' is a better role model. A psychosocial approach, they contend, is considerably more likely to be adopted by the nonpsychiatric physician if this role is modeled in an integrated approach to the patient by a 'medical liaisonist' than if it is recommended by a psychiatric consultant.

Recently, I was told by a friendly and perceptive internist that when working with house staff, people from psychiatry had an initial large obstacle to overcome before they walked on to the ward. This obstacle was the identification of such people as being from the department of psychiatry. House staff in internal medicine seem to be suspicious or mistrustful of psychiatrists. Such prejudice is also found among senior nonpsychiatric faculty who are training and role modeling for the house staff. The attitudes of these faculty towards psychiatry may have strong influences in determining the attitudes of house staff and medical students as described by *Nielson and Eaton* [1981]. They suggest that psychiatrists are taken more seriously if they demonstrate nonpsychiatric medical knowledge. In addition, there are methods of dealing with this prejudice [*Schubert*, 1978, 1979, 1980].

Once a nonpsychiatrist becomes convinced that psychiatry is legitimate and should be viewed as a part of the medical team treating the whole person, less ongoing reinforcement is required. Perhaps this is part of the reason for advocating the 'medical liaisonist': with the 'medical liaisonist' having identification with the nonpsychiatric department and at least some expertise or training in the nonpsychiatric specialty department, perhaps there is less initial suspicion of his motives and methods.

Unfortunately, the medical liaisonist may not have a comprehensive grasp of psychiatry if he is not a psychiatrist. How far then does the psychosocial basic knowledge of a medical liaisonist extend? One of the difficulties with current psychiatric consultation is that only a small percentage of people with psychiatric illnesses on nonpsychiatric wards are referred to the psychiatric consultant. Presumably, this could be an advantage of the 'medical liaisonist' who would be assigned full time to the unit and be thereby able to detect psychopathology which would ordinarily go unnoticed. Although this seems to be a potential advantage, it does not seem to be one of the major arguments advanced in favor of promulgating 'medical liaisonists'.

### Areas Where Psychiatric Consultant and 'Medical Liaisonist' Would Perform Differently

There are a number of areas where psychiatric consultants may perform differently from 'medical liaisonists'. In addition, there would be a number of areas where the effectiveness of a 'medical liaisonist' and that of the psychiatric consultant would be different because of their different roles. These are tendencies and should not be viewed as absolute differences. Some differences will be based on differences in personality and training within as well as between the groups.

Some areas where psychiatric consultants may have an advantage over 'medical liaisonists' would be in indirect consultation liaison [*Lowe* et al., 1971]. Indirect consultation is that consultation activity which involves either very little or no actual contact with the patient. This would involve helping the primary physician to care for the patient without intervening directly. Although this is not done by many consultants, the possibility would seem to be less likely for a 'medical liaisonist'. The 'medical liaisonist' as an integral part of the unit would see not only patients who he had been asked to see, but also other patients on a more routine basis who had not presented problems to date.

*Gunther* [1979] suggests that there is at times pathology in the group that results in consultation with the patient as the identified difficulty. He goes on to suggest that at times it is the overall group that has the difficulty and not the patient alone. This orientation of viewing the people on a medical ward as a group would seem more likely to come from a psychiatric consultant with more group training than from a 'medical liaisonist'. This group viewpoint would be one strategy in the indirect consultation.

Areas in which the 'medical liaisonist' would find it easier to work than a psychiatric consultant would be (a) where there are low referral rates [*Pritchard*, 1972], and (b) where patients voice a dislike of psychiatric referral [*Mezey and Kellett*, 1971]. Both of these areas may be dealt with by a psychiatric consultant who is also able to do some liaison. Methods of dealing with such difficulties will be examined in a later section.

Low referral rates were found by *Pritchard* [1972] to be particularly true in mental disorder, personality disorder, and alcoholism. *Houpt* et al. [1980] have found that usually only a small minority of patients with psychopathology are referred to a psychiatrist. Since a 'medical liaisonist' is assigned to a unit, access to patients who would not otherwise be referred is increased. This may overcome some of the difficulties of nonreferral.

*Mezey and Kellett* [1971] found that if a patient disliked the idea of a psychiatric referral, this would decrease the chances of the patient having such a referral. Since a 'medical liaisonist' would not be seeing the patient on psychiatric referral, this would be less of a problem for the 'medical liaisonist' than the consulting psychiatrist.

### Methods of Overcoming Difficulties with Consultation Psychiatry

*Schubert* [1978, 1979, 1980] has indicated in prior communications ways that obstacles to effective consultation liaison from a psychiatric point of view can be reduced or minimized. In an initial article [*Schubert*, 1978], the effectiveness of psychiatric consultation liaison was suggested to be increased by (1) acknowledging the primacy of care by nonpsychiatric colleagues; (2) avoiding direct as well as implied criticism for lack of psychiatric knowledge; (3) avoiding direct or implied diagnoses of nonpsychiatric physicians or other health personnel; (4) acknowledging the difficulty in dealing with patients with combined physical and psychiatric problems; (5) avoiding any unusual behavior that could be labeled 'eccentric'; (6) serving willingly and seriously in interdepartmental or interservice committees; (7) discussing collaborative research of an interdepartmental nature where there is a genuine interest, and (8) attending functions of medical staff in order to become known to others as well as to recognize and converse with nonpsychiatric physicians.

In a later article [*Schubert*, 1979], a further group of suggestions was made to increase the psychosocial sensitivity in nonpsychiatrists which may help reduce the problem with low referral rate. These included (1) accept referrals on difficult to get to or 'baffling' patients; (2) increase face-to-face meetings with potential consultees; (3) show nonpsychiatric physicians ongoing working formulations – this may help encourage both earlier referrals and joint management; (4) use consultation psychiatry to teach medical students and thereby show the relevance of psychosocial factors in nonpsychiatric settings; (5) help nonpsychiatric physicians with referral to other psychiatrists when the consulting psychiatrist is not able to take the patient, and (7) encourage explanation to the patient at all stages of evaluation and management in order to increase therapeutic regimen compliance.

In recent experience, it has been found useful for consulting psychiatry teams to arrange meetings with senior nonpsychiatric staff on a regular basis. This may be as infrequently as once a year. A formal office meeting has been found to be helpful. Preferably as indicated above, the consultant or consultants should have already met the senior nonpsychiatric staff before requesting this liaison meeting, through some of the methods suggested above. If not, this initial meeting proves valuable for this purpose as well. Psychiatrists can show their consultees their willingness to discuss problems relating to consultation, as well as showing their availability. They can demonstrate that they can talk in words understandable to the nonpsychiatrists. Such meetings should usually start with the departmental director or chairman, but do not end there. Consultants should then make attempts to meet with other unit directors and senior staff people. Frequently, this will serve as an arena to bring up other problems with the psychiatric department which are not directly related to consultation. The consultant, however, should continue to indicate availability and discuss with his chairman any serious and ongoing problems in the nonconsultation section of the psychiatry department.

In addition to meeting with senior staff people, psychiatric consultants should also meet with the chief nurse and at times other ward staff on each ward. It has frequently been useful for psychiatric consultants to attend rounds on the nonpsychiatric service. This will allow him to introduce himself to house staff physicians and other personnel involved on the consultee wards.

In teaching settings there is frequently not only rotation of house staff but also of senior teaching nonpsychiatric faculty. Psychiatric consultants should try to contact such visitants or attending physicians prior to the beginning of their rotation.

*Nielsen and Eaton* [1981] find that nonpsychiatric faculty frequently tell medical students that psychiatry is ineffective, unscientific, nonmedical, practiced by neurotics, emotionally overwhelming, and productive of high levels of career dissatisfaction. The consultant psychiatrist is the person with most contact with and therefore most likely to be able to dispel these myths among nonpsychiatrists. *Nielsen and Eaton* [1981] suggest drawing attention to the rigorously scientific and therapeutically effective aspects of psychiatry as well as specifically addressing the other myths. The consultant psychiatrist is most often the contact person and should bear a major burden of this work.

### How to Overcome Disadvantages of the 'Medical Liaisonist'

Since the 'medical liaisonist' term is perhaps newly introduced by this publication, little has been written specifically about it. Some of the potential or applied difficulties with a 'medical liaisonist' can be overcome by orientation and various types of additional training. Where the 'medical liaisonist' is a psychiatrist, areas covered in psychiatric residency are already known to him or her.

The 'medical liaisonist' may have many of the same difficulties as the psychiatric consultant. For example, it may be that the person talking of psychosocial difficulties may be thought of as a psychiatrist and therefore with suspicion. Thus, many of the methods mentioned above are applicable to the medical liaisonist as well as the psychiatric consultant. The use of language and words known primarily to psychiatrists should be avoided (as it should be with the psychiatrist consultant).

In other areas such as viewing the ward as a group, the 'medical liaisonist' may have more difficulty. This may be particularly difficult initially when deeply involved with such type of liaison. Perhaps serving as 'medical liaisonist' to several wards would be one method of gaining greater perspective on the ward.

The use of indirect liaison does not seem out of the purview of the 'medical liaisonist' as described by Lowe et al. [1971]. However, here again there may be pressure to see patients directly, particularly when the 'medical liaisonist' is a full-time member of the unit. Initially, this pressure should be dealt with by intermittent distancing.

Training other than a psychiatric residency for the task of 'medical liaisonist' may results in overemphasis on either ward management procedures or on psychoanalytic formulations. In the case of the former, there may be decreased emphasis on such traditional psychiatric illnesses such as schizophrenia and neuroses. Neuroses tend to be frequently overlooked as the patients with ward management problems tend to be the schizophrenics and personality disorders. Where primary care is an object, the quiet, compliant patient who is not a ward management problem but nevertheless has treatable psychopathology may not come to the attention of the primary care-giver. Those 'medical liaisonists' who receive little specific training in diagnosis and treatment of neurosis will be at a disadvantage in this area.

Similarly, those 'medical liaisonists' who receive little training in the management and treatment of schizophrenics will find this as a disadvantage in responding to schizophrenics on the ward. Nonpsychiatrists tend not to want to treat, manage, or be responsible for schizophrenics in their in-patient practices. The 'medical liaisonist' may be at a disadvantage if he is the only resource available at this point as this will result in the 'medical liaisonist' being responsible for the care of schizophrenics who are patients of non-psychiatrists as well. The procedure to overcome these difficulties in the 'medical liaisonists' training is to require greater experience in the diagnosis and treatment of neuroses and psychoses.

A second type of 'medical liaisonist' with which the writer is familiar is one who is not a psychiatrist but has had extensive psychoanalytic training. This is brought home in the fact that textbooks of medicine [*Wintrobe* et al., 1974] describe a functional diarrhea or irritable colon as having symptoms consistent with an anxiety neurosis. While this may at times be the case, many patients with such disorders do not meet the criteria for neurosis. Here the problem is the reverse of that presented in the preceding section: there is overemphasis on neurosis as being a prevailing cause of psychiatric disability in patients with nonpsychiatric illness who also seem to have medical diagnoses. The current *Diagnostic Manual III* [American Psychiatric Association, 1980] indicates a broad range of diagnoses that should be applied in various types of conditions in which physical symptoms are present and psychiatric diagnoses are appropriate. In addition, psychiatric problems presenting with physical symptoms are reviewed by *Lipowski* [1967]. Schizophrenia and stress disorders are associated with increased report of physical symptoms [*Hurst* et al., 1976]. A similar type of solution seems appropriate here in that the 'medical liaisonist' should have a broad background in psychiatry including psychotic disorders, somatoform disorders, personality disorders, and adjustment reactions.

*Conclusions*

The 'medical liaisonist' is a physician with his primary identification in a department other than psychiatry and with at least some training in a department other than psychiatry. The consultant psychiatrist, on the other hand, retains his identity as a psychiatrist and is not a full-time member of a nonpsychiatric department. One of the clear differences implied from the differences in definition is that the 'liaisonist' would be subjected to less prejudice against psychiatrists, although there might be some prejudice as a result of frequent emphasis on psychosocial issues. The 'medical liaisonist' would also have an advantage of being more likely to come in contact with patients who may have psychosocial problems but would not receive a formal psychiatric consultation.

The 'medical liaisonist' who does not have psychiatric training may find the disadvantage of misunderstanding of some areas of diagnosis and treatment in psychiatry to be a considerable disadvantage. A further disadvantage with the 'medical liaisonist' may be the difficulty in viewing patient-physician-other staff together as a group. A number of areas of potential differences are not clear from the definition and probably would differ within the 'liaisonist' group and within consultant psychiatrists.

As a group there are a number of ways of overcoming difficulties of the consultant psychiatrist, a number of which can be grouped into increased liaison functions. The psychiatrist must be approachable and plain speaking. Usefulness is desirable both in formulation and management as well in practical matters such as finding a psychiatric disposition. Finally, consultant psychiatrists should perhaps, as part of their liaison function, meet with nonpsychiatric department directors, unit chiefs, and head nurses on a regular basis.

Ways are also suggested to overcome some of the disadvantages of the 'medical liaisonist'. Since there is some overlap in roles between the 'medical liaisonist' and the consultant psychiatrist, some of the difficulties may be overcome by ways suggested for the consultant psychiatrist. This would include overcoming the distrust of people who give psychosocial advice or are otherwise especially psychiatrically oriented. The 'medical liaisonist' may overcome deep involvement in a ward or unit by separating himself from it for at least brief periods. If the 'medical liaisonist' is not a psychiatrist, training in all areas of diagnosis and management of mental illness will help overcome deficiencies in total psychiatric management capabilities.

The differences between the 'medical liaisonist' and the psychiatric consultant thus can frequently be overcome where there are disadvantages. It seems to the author that the outlook for the future is that the general field of medicine will require as many consultant psychiatrists as well as many 'medical liaisonists' as make themselves available to such positions. While people in each role should keep in touch with those in the other role and thereby enhance their usefulness, it does not seem to the author that there will be any practical difficulty between the two groups. Serving the clinical functions of either the consultant psychiatrist, particularly with liaison included, or the 'medical liaisonist' will be more than enough for anyone to do. Thus, it is hoped that other areas of medicine will come to understand the usefulness of both roles and encourage their employment in academic and nonacademic departments both of psychiatry and other medical fields.

## References

American Psychiatric Association: Diagnostic and statistical manual of mental disorders; 3rd ed. (Washington 1980).

Engel, G.L.: Presentation at 1980 American Psychosomatic Society Meeting.

Gunther, M.S.: The psychopathology of psychiatric consultation. A different view. Comp. Psychiat. *20:* 187–198 (1979).

Houpt, J.L.; Orleans, C.S.; George, L.K.; Brodie, H.K.H.: The role of psychiatric and behavioral factors in the practice of medicine. Am. J. Psychiat. *137:* 37–47 (1980).

Hurst, M.W.; Jenkins, C.D.; Rose, R.M.: Relationship of psychological stress to onset of medical illness. A. Rev. Med. *27:* 301–312 (1976).

Lipowski, Z.J.: Review of consultation psychiatry and psychosomatic medicine. II. Clinical aspects. Psychosom. Med. *29:* 201–224 (1967).

Lowe, D.J.; et al.: Problems in achieving indirect psychiatric consultation. Hosp. Commun. Psychiat. *22:* 91–94 (1971).

Mezey, A.G.; Kellett, J.M.: Reasons against referral to the psychiatrist. Post-grad. med. J. *47:* 315 (1971).

Nielsen, A.C. III; Eaton, J.S., Jr.: Medical students' attitudes about psychiatry. Archs gen. Psychiat. *38:* 1144–1154 (1981).

Pritchard, M.: Who sees a psychiatrist? A study of factors related to psychiatric referral in the general hospital. Post-grad. med. J. *48:* 456–461 (1972).

Reichsman, F.: Teaching psychosomatic medicine to medical students, residents and postgraduate fellows. Int. J. psychiat. Med. *5:* 589–598 (1974).

Schubert, D.S.P.: Obstacles to effective psychiatric liaison. Psychosomatics *19:* 283–285 (1978).

Schubert, D.S.P.: How the liaison psychiatrist can improve his usefulness. Psychiat. Annls *9:* 36–38 (1979).

Schubert, D.S.P.: Improving the effectiveness of consultation by psychiatrists and from psychiatrists. J. psychiat. Treatm. Eval. *2:* 111–113 (1980).

Wintrobe, M.D.; Thorn, G.W.; Adams, R.D.; Braunwald, E.; Isselbacher, K.J.; Petersdorf, R.G.: Harrison's principles of internal medicine; 7th ed. (McGraw-Hill, New York 1974).

D. Schubert, MD, PhD, Case Western Reserve University School of Medicine, and Cleveland Metropolitan General Hospitals, Cleveland, OH 44106 (USA)

# Clinical Activities throughout the World

Adv. psychosom. Med., vol. 11, pp. 62–73 (Karger, Basel 1983)

# Consultation-Liaison Psychiatry in Panama

*Rafael Sabonge[a], Ovidio A. De León[b], Jaime Arroyo[c]*

[a] Santo Tomás Hospital, Department of Medicine and University of Panama
School of Medicine; [b] Psychiatric Services, Santo Tomás Hospital and
Santa María University School of Psychology; [c] Santo Tomás Hospital and
University of Panama School of Medicine, Panama City, Panama

## Historical Note

The history of consultation-liaison psychiatry in Panama is closely linked to the emergence of general hospital psychiatry. It was not until 1971 that the service of psychiatry was organized at Santo Tomás Hospital, the largest and oldest medical institution in the Republic of Panama. Prior to that, a psychiatrist did consultation to medical and surgical wards as well as directing an outpatient psychiatric clinic organized around the traditional medical model. At that time, the hospital lacked the services of psychologists, psychiatric nurses, and psychiatric social workers. Within this context, the work of the psychiatrist was limited to assist in the treatment of patients designated as 'mental cases' and his impact in teaching and handling psychosocial factors was negligible. Although administratively within the Department of Medicine, the psychiatrist was actually perceived as an outside consultant and was never integrated into departmental work, not even in the role of a psychosomaticist.

Psychiatric services provided at Santo Tomás Hospital before 1971 were a small portion of the services rendered by the psychiatric care system as a whole. The system had been limited for many years to the National Psychiatric Hospital, a large, understaffed, overpopulated, custodial institution. The model of psychiatry known to the medical community was derived from attending psychiatric undergraduate courses taught at that freestanding hospital. By the end of the 1960s, encouraged by changing societal values, young psychiatrists became dissatisfied by this state of affairs and initiated modifications that resulted in the development of new models for psychiatric services. Panamanian psychiatry did not escape the influences described by

*Talbott* [1] in determining the delivery of psychiatric services. The pressures that brought about the opening of the in-patient psychiatric unit at Santo Tomás Hospital came from the National Psychiatric Hospital. The opening of such a unit was opposed by influential medical leaders at Santo Tomás, but their objections were overriden by the Ministry of Health. Unfortunately, the general hospital unit was initially under administrative control of the National Psychiatric Hospital. This arrangement became a nidus of conflict due to the double line of authority. The quality of patient care and the development of effective liaison efforts were hindered due to this structural format. In 1979, Santo Tomás Hospital took over full administrative responsibility of the psychiatric services, allowing the development of a broad range of innovative services.

In summary, psychiatric services within Panama have evolved from freestanding asylums to satellites within general medical settings to the present situation of an integrated general hospital psychiatric unit. Our general psychiatric unit is now under the administrative direction of psychiatrists who report to the hospital medical staff, not to the national psychiatric hospital administration. From this 'island of psychiatry' within a general medical setting, a nucleus of individuals coalesced and developed liaison activities. The chairman of the Department of Medicine, Dr. *Sabonge*, is a gastroenterologist who has long been interested in the psychosocial aspects of medical practice. 7 years ago, he spent a sabbatical year in liaison psychiatry with Dr. *Lipowski*. Returning from this experience, he has been instrumental in providing the administrative support and intellectual encouragement to develop such a liaison program. Psychiatrists involved in early liaison efforts included Dr. *Arroyo* who had been influenced by psychoanalysis during his training in Argentina and was interested in preventive psychiatry following completion of a masters in public health from Johns Hopkins University. Finally, the senior author was influenced in psychosomatic medicine while training in Peru under Dr. *Carlos Seguin*, the famed psychosomaticist. During residency training at the University of Maryland, he was also able to participate and observe the effects of an active liaison service.

The efforts to implement a liaison service at Santo Tomás started in 1975 when a weekly clinical conference was established as part of the regular teaching activities of the Department of Medicine [2]. It was around this conference that psychosocial factors began to be taught and doctors started to feel the need to identify and manage them in all types of physical illnesses, in order to promote the optimal care of their patients. A good indicator of the effectiveness of this approach was the steady increase of consultations that went up by 122% from 1974 to 1980.

During this time, the hospital medical staff began to realize that the Psychiatry Division lacked the organizational structure to provide sorely needed services without available consultants. This lack of structure was clearly related to the double line of authority in the psychiatric unit as well as the lack of commitment of traditional psychiatrists to the liaison work. At this point the hospital medical and psychiatric staff collaborated to obtain the funds needed to take full responsibility of the psychiatric services. Thus, the most important consequence of the initial efforts of the consultation work was to bring about the administrative changes needed to develop a psychiatric service independent of the National Psychiatric Hospital. In turn, this paved the way for a more comprehensive liaison program.

The history of our liaison work occurred in three stages. The first was the stage of consultation performed by a psychiatrist working as a 'solo' practitioner. The second was the beginning of liaison work, and the third is the fully developed consultation-liaison service. The efforts of traditional psychiatrists were important to move from the first to the second phase, but they did not prove to be committed to the idea of liaison work. They were too near sighted and their notion of general hospital psychiatry was limited to the transplantation of a custodial ward into the general hospital. In order to move from the second to the third stage it was pivotal to influence the medical and surgical staff already sensitized to the benefits of liaison work. It is important to note at this point that there is no other fully developed psychiatric liaison work in the country. Our efforts, errors and trials are therefore important models in the path that other hospitals will have to follow in our country, and probably in other developing countries as well.

### The Scope of Our Activities

The Service of Psychiatry is organizationally within the Department of Medicine. It is therefore specifically designated and integrated into the rest of the hospital's activities. From the structural point of view, the service is organized around four different areas: in-patient care, outpatient care, emergency services, and liaison-consultation. The in-patient unit is a 24-bed, voluntary, open door facility, with an active milieu program and an eclectic therapeutic approach. The average length of stay is 23 days, and 370 admissions were handled in 1980. The outpatient services had 3,084 visits in the same year. It is noteworthy that our clinic for affective disorders manages 90 bipolar patients who receive lithium treatment. It is here that depressed patients are routinely evaluated and treated. This is the clinical arena for an active team effort, including nephrologists and endocrinologists. Our emergency service evaluates 2% of incoming cases using a team approach and crisis intervention techniques including up to 72 h emergency hospitalization. In 1980, 768 patients were seen by the crisis team in the emergency room. The psychiatric staff consists of 3 full-time psychiatrists, 1 part-time psychiatrist, 2 clinical psychologists, 1 psychiatric social worker, 7 psychiatric nurses, and 3 psychiatric aides. Residents from the National Psychiatric Hospital spend a 6-month rotation on the in-patient unit and they can elect to spend an additional 2 months in our liaison program. Santo Tomás Hospital has its own psychiatric residency program which includes a 12-month rotation in liaison psychiatry. The psychiatric staff includes people with strong biologic preference as well as clinicians with a marked psychodynamic orientation, giving our work a truly eclectic flavor. Less emphasis is placed on behavioristic interventions, but some biofeedback techniques are used on selected cases for teaching purposes. We have no space on the medical areas of the hospital and we use our own space for family interviews and follow-up visits. Space on medical areas, nonetheless, is used for clinical conferences, and patients' meetings, specifically diabetics, alcoholics, chronic dialysis and cancer patients.

Two psychiatrists are currently doing liaison work half time. One of them works exclusively with oncology patients and the other takes care of the rest of the hospital. Our second year resident works 12 months on liaison and devotes approximately 70% of his time to it. The rest of the time is spent doing long-term and short-term outpatient psychotherapy. The social worker and the psychologists participate in the evaluation of selected cases and help in their management too. The psychologists have also been participating in the research endeavors now in progress. Our psychiatric nurses have been instrumental in developing a continuing training course in clinical communication for nurses and aides, which is regarded highly by the participants. In addition to this they are doing liaison work with chronic dialysis patients and their families. No one is doing full-time exclusive liaison work. But almost everybody in the service is in some way connected with our liaison efforts. Thus, there is a great deal of interest and commitment in the psychiatric staff for tightening up our relationships with the rest of the hospital.

Our liaison work with oncology is only a few months old. It was first directed toward establishing a working relationship with the doctors by attending clinical rounds and clinical conferences. Some patients were seen directly, but the emphasis was placed in understanding how the system operated, evaluating what the needs were and trying to develop a list of priorities. We found it easier to work in radiotherapy. The facilities were surveyed, the patients fears were assessed, and the work routines were observed. The information gathered in this way enabled us to make some recommendations about changes in the physical environment and changes in the work routines that have impact in the patients' psychological reactions to the procedures. Once the patients fears were assessed and understood, we met with the radiation technicians. As a result, some changes in the physical environment took place and the patients started to receive information about the equipment and the meaning of noises and movements that previously was seldom explained to them. We are now trying to extend experiences like this to the area of chemotherapy, as well as other outpatient and in-patient areas. The strategy is to work with nursing and technical staff in order to sensitize them to the patients' psychological needs. We expect to have a wider impact in the quality of patient care using this approach instead of emphasizing individual care. We are also now planning group meetings with breast cancer and gynecological cancer patients with the purpose of producing cognitive and affective changes in these patients toward their illnesses.

Our alcoholism services are integrated in our liaison work too. Alcoholic patients in medical-surgical wards are invited to participate in the program for alcoholics hospitalized in the psychiatric unit. In this way we can save staff time and make the experience more relevant to all alcoholics involved.

The development of our residency program was geared at providing the opportunity for an intensive exposure to liaison work. We feel that this is one of the most important areas of expertise that psychiatrists have to develop in our country if we really want to take psychiatry out of its isolation in the asylum. The 2nd-year resident spends 12 months rotating in different areas of medicine and neurology-neurosurgery. During this rotation the resisdent is given specific clinical assignments which he has to carry out jointly with the resident in internal medicine. In addition to that, he has to answer consultations from surgical, medical, oncological and obstetrics-gynecological wards. He is also actively involved in the research efforts going on in the liaison service. This experience is highly valued when the child psychiatry year rotation is taken up. The psychiatric resident's role in our program includes participation in the nonpsychiatric service's work, generation of consultations, evaluations for all patients for whom consultation is requested, participation in clinical conferences about comprehensive patient care, organization and coordination of lectures and seminars and, finally, the opportunity to pursue research interests. The resident's schedule allows for limited outpatient follow-up. At present, our service lacks separate organizational divisions, but we hope to move in that direction. This lack of structure, however, provides no conflicts in the resident's supervision. Residents from the National Psychiatric Hospital rotating in our service have shown little interest, with some exceptions, in our liaison work, probably because the reasons which attracted them to psychiatry as a specialty have little to do with the practice of medicine.

### The Health Delivery System: Boundaries, Articulation and Conflict

The Panamanian health delivery system is divided into two sectors: public and private. We do not include the folkloric net of health care, which is an exceedingly important source of care for thousands of patients. The discussion of this sector is out of the scope of this paper. The public health sector can be subdivided into the social security subsystem and the public health subsystem. The social security subsystem is responsible for providing health care, retirement and other benefits to all workers and their immediate family members in the country. Over the past 10 years this sector has increased its population coverage due to the progressive liberalization of the laws governing its operation. As a consequence, the quality of care provided by this sector has been deteriorating, and many of these patients go into the public health or the private sectors for assistance.

The public health subsystem is responsible for providing health care and preventive services to the entire population. Public health institutions find themselves increasingly encumbered financially by the admission of patients who receive emergency care in social security hospitals and are subsequently transferred to public health hospitals for additional treatment. There are also patients who perceive social security institutions as too bureaucratic and seek medical services in the public health sector. Services provided to these patients are not reimbursed to public health institutions. Over the past few years an integration of the two subsystems has been pursued and accomplished partially, but no improvement in the quality of care has been noticed in either sector, leaving the door open to intense criticism regarding the wisdom of these policies.

The decline of the public sector as the primary provider of services affects the delivery of services in the private sector. At present, the private sector handles 5% of the total bed capacity in the country and this figure is slowly increasing. The growth of in-patient private facilities is difficult by the high cost of medical services and high interest rates that make investment in health care expensive. Private medicine is practiced along a continuum line having at one end extremely well-equipped and staffed medical centers, and, at the other end, popular clinics where substandard care is the rule. Psychiatry is represented in the entire spectrum, but even at the more affluent end there are no adequate in-patient psychiatric facilities. There is only one private psychiatric hospital in the country which is merely custodial. In reference to funding in private consultation-liaison psychiatry, insurance carriers, probably assuming that physicians might engage in fee splitting and cross-referrals do not pay psychiatric consultants their appropriate fees.

Santo Tomás Hospital belongs to the public health subsystem. General hospital psychiatry, including liaison-consultation, shares a number of problems with the institution as a whole. Funding problems, for example, affects psychiatry just as well as other specialties, along the boundaries between the public health sector and the social security sector. But in addition to that, general hospital psychiatry has to deal with internal boundaries within the public health sector. Psychiatric services at Santo Tomás have to compete for funds with the National Psychiatric Hospital, and in this regard it has been very frustrating to see that five times more residents are allocated to the psychiatric hospital than to Santo Tomás Hospital, in spite of a more progressive and complete training program at our hospital.

A conceptual confluct within the public health subsystem of psychiatric services limits the growth of liaison psychiatry. On the one hand, psychiatrists from the National Psychiatric Hospital and the Department of Mental Health of the Ministry of Health are committed to a biological model of psychiatry in an overly simplistic way. The allocation of money and resources is decided in favor of institutions and programs that conform to this custodial-biological approach. On the other hand, we advocate at Santo Tomás Hospital the adoption of a holistic view that unifies all the multidimensional factors that play a role in psychiatric illness and treatment. We can think of no other way in which consultation with other medical disciplines can take place.

The resolution of these conflicts will have a most profound repercussion in the future of Panamanian psychiatry. We believe that planning that originates within the hospital structure has the best chance to be adequate and relevant. This is why we resist external directives not in tune with our own clinical base. But we also understand that planning that comes from superordinated structures is also needed if the general hospital is to be functionally linked with other facilities within the psychiatric system network. We are now trying strategies that will enable us to maintain our integrity while we participate and coordinate actions with the rest of the system. We also understand that many times the allocation of monies is decided following intense political and social pressures and not rational health planning. A process of negotiated intersystem and intrasystem planning will have to take place in order to delineate our role in the psychiatric service system [3].

### Learners and Learning

Usually, the primary focus of educational efforts in medicine has been upon medical students. The University of Panama School of Medicine unfortunately lacks a university hospital. Medical students go to Santo Tomás Hospital and Social Security Hospital for their clinical rotations. They also go to rural general hospitals and health outposts when appropriate. They are still going to the National Psychiatric Hospital for their clinical rotation, emphasizing in this way only one model of psychiatry. When they come out of that rotation their uniformly negative regard for psychiatry is rather striking. The contact with our established liaison program during their internal medicine clerkship helps many of them to change their negative evaluation of psychiatry and psychosomatic medicine, as well as to learn about the importance of psychological and social factors in health and illness.

We try to involve all hospital staff in some learning experience relevant to the psychosocial needs of the patient. Different methods have been employed, including lectures, seminars, clinical conferences, clinical rounds, staff group dynamics and direct supervision. Nonpsychiatric specialists have been less involved in these organized activities, but not less interested. Time factors become a major obstacle. House staff involved in formal and informal teaching activities have shown a great deal of interest. The department of medicine has established a month rotation in psychiatry for their residents, which is to be taken during their second or third year of training. Interns are also offered an elective rotation in psychiatry. The psychiatric residents have been both students and educators and find the experience highly formative. Nurses and aides are welcomed to attend lectures and case presentations as well as participate in the continuing courses on clinical communication given by the psychiatric nurses.

We have always been concerned about how to make more rational use of professional time, particularly in the light of our very scarce resources. It is very important for us to accomplish the right balance between the time spent in direct patient care and the time devoted to meeting the educational needs of the hospital staff. In our experience each service is at a different level in terms of its educational needs and its capacity to assimilate our help. We have found that system analysis is the best way to assess the needs of a particular area of the hospital. We conceptualize services in our hospital as located along a continuum line having at one extreme services with strong leadership, tight organizational structures, low conflict tolerance and low staff turnover (type A), and at the other end services characterized by weak leadership, frequently changing regulations, high staff turnover, and high levels of conflict that reverberate throughout the entire system and even have extrasystem repercussions (type Z). In the first type of units, we found that even a small educational effort usually had a long-lasting impact on the quality of patient care and the staff developed confidence and skills in handling emotional problems without our direct help. Units situated at the other end find it more difficult to make use of an educational approach and have to spend more time in direct patient care. Type A units sometimes start out with very low levels of psychological sophistication, but once some changes take place, they are maintained by the homeostatic mechanisms of the system. Type Z units very frequently can do nothing but waste the skills of very sophisticated staff members. In other words, sociological characteristics are the best predictors of the type of involvement that we will develop with other services. The dilemma in working with type Z units is to play or not to play a complementary relationship. In either case the results are expected to be poor and our time effort will not be compensated by some lasting changes. Probably the answer to this dilemma is to help type Z units to move toward the A end of the scale, but that will move us away from the traditional role of a liaison worker and will represent a challenge in time and political effort that we are not prepared to take.

We can briefly illustrate some of our teaching experiences in liaison work.

The opening of the intensive care burn unit took place after careful planning that emphasized infection control. The psychiatrists' views were not asked and the nursing staff had no previous experience in these types of units. The result was the construction of a sensory deprivation chamber. Every patient admitted to this unit during the first 3 months of operation developed intense psychiatric reactions, ranging from severe depressions to acute delirium. We took this as an opportunity to discuss with the staff some of the issues involved. Some changes in the physical environment and work routines took place and the nursing staff gradually became sensitive and skilled in handling the psychosocial dimensions of these patients.

The intensive care coronary unit, as opposed to the burn unit, was very well designed in terms of its physical environment and the psychological needs of the patients. Nurses and aides were carefully selected and trained. Shortly after the opening of the unit conflict erupted between staff members. We were called in consultation and after an initial evaluation it was agreed to have a weekly meeting with the nursing staff. The director of the unit was scheduled to attend these meetings fortnightly, and the objective was to explore the interpersonal tensions arising in this type of work. Nurses began exploring the tensions in the interface between house staff officers and them, but conflicts in this area were only a reflection of an irrational fear arising in the light of their intense competition. They were concerned about who was going to be working at the time of the first death in the unit. As we continued exploring this issue it became evident that this intense sibling rivalry originated from the strong paternalistic attitude that the unit's director displayed toward them. Once these feelings were resolved the tension diminished and they continued working as a team with the high level of competence expected from them.

Infectious disease specialists are particularly aware of the psychiatric complications of their patients. They work closely with us and have included in their team a nurse with training in both infectious disease and psychiatry. There was a disagreement between plastic surgeons from the burn unit and internists about the use of antibiotics. In some instances this disagreement interfered with the proper care of the patients. The psychiatric nurse has played an important role on those occasions, helping to negotiate an agreement between the parties involved, under our supervision.

The above clinical examples show how teaching and service cannot be separated. In many instances, we have defined differential objectives in reference to our potential learners and we use different educational experiences to meet the needs of different health personnel in various settings. In spite of that, the main obstacle that we are facing is the lack of psychiatrists' time. We feel that we are overextended and can no longer meet the growing demands of liaison activities.

Finally, patients are also potential learners. In this area we have gained some experience in our clinic for affective disorders and in the treatment of diabetic outpatients. We are now developing video techniques in order to improve our effectiveness in this area.

## *Collaborative Strategies for Research in Consultation-Liaison Psychiatry*

At Santo Tomás Hospital we are lucky to have a medical staff heavily committed to the idea of comprehensive patient care, and a psychiatric staff equally devoted to the notion of holistic medicine. Once this is said, it is known that we have to deal only with external obstacles and funding problems. The same is not true for other hospitals in the country.

In this environment it is easy to find common ground for research interests. We first became interested in studying our suicide attempters in relation to stressful life events. We developed a research design that required a control group of medical patients, and after talking about the idea with the gastroenterologists, they offered their collaboration in this endeavor. We were able to interview 61 patients from the gastroenterology outpatient clinic and the results are now being analyzed. Secondly, the endocrinology section showed interest in our help to work with their diabetic patients. They have managed to organize an Association of Diabetic Patients that meets regularly for educational purposes and social gatherings. They wanted to have our expertise in groups at their disposal, as well as our help in individual cases. We worked together for a while and soon a research project took form. We were interested to study the relationship between life stress and diabetic control and developed a design that included a retrospective and a prospective study. The diabetic control is being assessed by the determination of glycosylate hemoglobin which as far as we know has never been used in a study like this. The retrospective study is now completed and the results are under statistical analysis. The prospective study is currently in progress. At this point it is important to note that research money is extremely tight in Panama. Our diabetes study has been partially funded by the patients themselves through their Association. We regard this as a most unique and rewarding development.

Our clinic for affective disorders is really a joint venture with endocrinologists and nephrologists as well. We are now performing dexamethasone suppression tests to our depressed patients with the help of the endocrinological laboratory, and expect to report our experience in the near future. Our lithium patients are routinely evaluated by endocrinologists and nephrologists and a report on this is also forthcoming.

As a result of our involvement with the medical-surgical wards we were invited to contribute a chapter in a multiauthored book on oncology [4].

The latest development in the area of research in liaison psychiatry is a project on the consequences of teenage pregnancy and delivery, which is also a collaborative effort by the Department of Obstetrics and Gynecology, the Service of Psychiatry, the School of Psychology of Santa María University and the Panamanian Association for Family Planning. This project has just been funded by the Agency for International Development. The goal of the study is to determine the psychosocial needs of adolescent mothers and their babies in order to develop relevant programs, anchored in our own reality.

The important common denominator of our research endeavors is collaboration. In all of them we look for a multidisciplinary cooperation with other services around areas that they regard as important and we can help with our resources and expertise. This approach has contributed to effectively integrate psychiatric and medical services.

We have demonstrated in Panama that the idea of liaison psychiatry is viable, even with scarce resources. The Panamanian Psychiatric Association is organizing a 2-day course on the 'Psychiatric Aspects of Medical Care', mainly for nonpsychiatric physicians, and the forthcoming annual meeting of the association will be devoted to liaison psychiatry. Santo Tomás medical staff will be heavily involved in both events. We look forward to them with the hope that they will become important milestones in the improvement of patient care and physician education in holistic medicine [5].

### References

1   Talbott, J.A.: The death of the asylum. A critical study of state hospital management, services and care (Grune & Stratton, New York 1978).
2   Sabonge, R.; De León, O.; Berroa, I.: Grupo médico-psiquiátrico del Hospital Santo Tomás. Revta méd. Panamá 2: 213–217 (1977).
3   Bachrach, L.L.: General hospital psychiatry. Overview from a sociological perspective. Am. J. Psychiat. 138: 879–887 (1981).
4   De León., O.: Oncología y Psiquiatría; in Avilés, Fuentes, Valdés, Young, Oncología básica, pp. 553–579 (Editorial Universitaria de Panamá, Panama 1981).
5   Lipowski, Z.J.: Holistic-medical foundations of American psychiatry. A bicentennial. Am. J. Psychiat. 138: 888–895 (1981).

R. Sabonge, MD, Santo Tomás Hospital, Department of Medicine,
University of Panama School of Medicine, Panama City (Panama)

Adv. psychosom. Med., vol. 11, pp. 74–87 (Karger, Basel 1983)

# Consultation-Liaison Psychiatry in Poland

*Zdzislaw Ryn*

Department of Psychiatry, Medical Academy in Kraków
(Director: Prof. *A. Szymusik*), Krakow, Poland

Polish psychiatry has a character of its own and is rooted in the old culture, tradition and Slavonic anthropology. Nevertheless, its research aspect has been shaped under the influence of German and British psychiatry. Despite a fairly homogeneous social and ideological structure of Polish society, psychiatry in Poland is diverse, sometimes eclectic. In some centers of medical care it is clearly biologically focused, while others dynamically or humanistically oriented. Different faces of Polish psychiatry are most probably the expression that Poles possess a natural need for liberty, independence and tolerance. The level of psychiatric culture in Polish society also varies, ranging from the view that mental disturbances demonstrate the latent possibilities of the evolution of the human psyche, to the stance that a mentally ill individual should be treated an outcast unworthy of any human rights.

This diversity is also reflected in consultation-liaison psychiatry, a subspecialty not isolated as an independent section of psychiatry, yet constitutes one of the most important links between clinical psychiatry and other disciplines of practical medicine.

Originally the role of consultants for the mental patients belonged to neuropsychiatrists since these two specialties remained together until the 1920s. So-called 'consylium' used to be held in those days and a neuropsychiatrist was sometimes invited. Up to World War II in Polish hospitals and university clinics these two specializations were combined. Although the oldest Department of Psychiatry was set up in 1905 in Krakow, the clinic, however, bore the name of the Neuro-psychiatric Clinic of the Jagiellonian University till after the war. In the 1950s psychiatric departments of the University became independent and have been functioning as such up till now. The majority of Polish hospitals and university clinics are behaviorally or psychodynamically oriented. Consultative psychiatry and psychosomatic medicine in Poland has its beginning in the second half of the 1950s.

## Mental Patients and Psychiatrists in Poland

The number of patients under ambulatory psychiatric care has reached the level of about half a million people per year (the population of Poland is now 36 million inhabitants). The most numerous group comprises neurotic patients (34.3%) and psychotic patients (31.3%), schizophrenic patients included (13.9%). The percentage of mentally retarded patients amounts to 6.5%. The intake of patients into psychiatric hospitals has recently increased up to 4/1,000 inhabitants. In the last decade the frequency of occurrence of alcoholic, senile and sclerotic psychoses has increased. The incidence of schizophrenia is tending to decrease, which may be the result of improvement in diagnostic methods. Among nonpsychotic disturbances, alcoholism, neuroses and drug addiction have grown. Suicidal attempts constitute the second most common cause of death in men at the age of 15–34, and in women at the age of 15–29. Concurrently mental disturbances in 1974 were the fourth cause of invalidism.

Within a province (Poland is divided into 49 administrative provinces) psychiatric care is delivered by psychiatric departments (hospital-based), or by the provincial mental health ambulatory, and by psychiatric hospitals (or psychiatric units). This is further supported by psychiatric clinics of Medical Academies (12 clinics). For the whole country psychiatric care is supervised by the Psychoneurological Institute in Warsaw.

Ambulatory care service has at its disposal 518 mental health clinics and 50 daily wards of altogether 1,300 places. There are 92 hospitals and psychiatric departments in Poland which gives the total number of 42,000 beds, i.e. 11.9/10,000 inhabitants. Psychiatric beds constitute 16% of the total number of all hospital beds. But they are mostly concentrated in 19 large hospitals of over 1,000 beds each. Social welfare homes of all types have at disposal 60,000 beds, half of which are occupied by people suffering from chronic mental diseases.

The number of qualified psychiatrists is approximately 1,700 physicians, i.e. 3.7% of the general number of physicians. This gives 4.6 psychiatrists/ 100,000 inhabitants. On average 1 physician has 32 hospital beds under his care. 400 psychologists are employed in psychiatric hospitals, 140 social assistants, 500 occupational therapy instructors, and nearly 300 special education teachers.

In 1979 about 2 million ambulatory consultations were delivered (59/ 1,000 inhabitants), and 145,000 patients hospitalized (410/100,000 inhabitants). The average period of treatment has been shortened in the last decade from 118 to 39 days. The tasks facing consultative psychiatry are continually growing since a number of indirect forms of care of mentally sick has been developing, such as day hospitals, rehabilitation centers, home hospitalization, hostels, psychiatric night wards, etc. It should be emphasized that all forms of medical care in Poland are welfare services and are free for the majority of inhabitants.

### The Consultant Psychiatrist and the Scope of His Tasks

Despite numerous official declarations acknowledging psychiatry to be one of basic and equal to other disciplines of medicine, in many countries, as well as in Poland, it still seems that 'psychiatry is the unwanted child of medicine'. Setting up psychiatric units in general hospitals has been recommended by psychiatrists for many years. Unfortunately, psychiatric beds in general hospitals make up only 10% of all psychiatric beds in Poland. Apart from their own medical work, general hospital units can perform special tasks resulting from the possibility of direct cooperation with other physicians. In a situation like this the psychiatrists can become a liaison consultant for other units of the hospital. Thus general hospital psychiatry seems to be the best model of integrating psychiatry with other disciplines of medicine.

Polish psychiatrists have already devoted considerable attention to this problem, though their postulates are still awaiting full realization [*Falicki*, 1967; *Wilczkowski*, 1952; *Wardaszko-Lyskowska*, 1971b]. The consultant psychiatrist within the Polish health service system occupies a special position and fulfills special functions. Clinical psychiatry has been and still is little known among physicians in general. A mentally ill patient arouses fear and provokes the family and the general physicians aiming to isolate this person in a psychiatric hospital as quickly as possible.

The structure and organization of the medical system in Poland creates favorable conditions for comprehensive development of consultative and liaison psychiatry, but the manner in which these possibilities will be realized depends on psychiatrists themselves, i.e. their clinical expertise as well as on their own personality and ability to secure the support of general physicians.

The duties of a consultant psychiatrist should normally be entrusted to a physician who is an experienced clinical psychiatrist, and who – at the same time – is sufficiently acquainted with practical general medicine. This helps to avoid certain errors such as directing patients with mental disturbances to psychiatric hospital while – in the first place – they demand intensive somatic treatment [*Jaska*, 1976].

The arena of psychiatric consultations in Poland is fairly extensive and apart from medicine itself, it covers such areas as schools, universities, state and social institutions, industry, judicature, family guidance, activity of priests and many others. In Poland consultative psychiatry is most frequently interpreted according to the criteria given by *Lipowski* [1967, 1968, 1971, 1974], i.e. as the branch of psychiatry which deals with diagnostic, therapeutic, didactic and research work of psychiatrists in general hospitals. It seems that the weakest point of Polish consultative psychiatry is that its didactic potentialities are not being exploited. There are few more ideal opportunities to show – on concrete, practical examples – a holistic, humanistic, dynamic psychosomatic approach to the patient and his illness. In addition, the consultant can help the staff to understand the patient's behavior and emotions, as well as the staff's own reactions and attitudes [*Wardaszko-Lyskowska*, 1971a].

Insufficient attention is paid to qualifications, personality characteristics and training of consultant psychiatrists. The consultant psychiatrist should be endowed with the 'third ear', i.e. he should be sensitive to symbolic meaning of behavior, recognize nonverbal and nonconscious material, should be able to establish interpersonal contacts easily, and have the ability to assist the team in charge of treatment in a tactful, unimposing manner.

Whatever the attitude of other physicians in a particular environment towards the consultant psychiatrist is, it is molded in the same way towards psychiatrists in general. This makes the role of a consultant exceptionally important, not only because of its medical aspect, but also because other physicians accept cooperation with psychiatry often because of a positive interaction with a consultant psychiatrist.

*Psychiatric Consultations in Medical Academies*
*(Some Model Solutions)*

In medical academies in Poland a practice has been adopted that experienced assistants of psychiatric clinics are simultaneously employed as liaison psychiatrists in other clinics, and hospital units. Thus the consultant psychiatrist gradually becomes a member of the diagnostic-therapeutic team. This close and permanent cooperation with the physician in charge of treatment of the patient makes it possible to solve not only biological but also psychosocial problems of the patient. The patient's needs after he has left the hospital are also covered. Within our medical care system this form of consultation is positively appraised by consultant psychiatrists themselves as well as by physicians who refer to it. Establishing liaison psychiatrists has enabled other physicians to achieve a better grasp of the role and scope of psychiatric help, made clear the purposefulness of engaging this help, and created optimum conditions for examination.

At the Medical Academy in Warsaw consultations had a rather sporadic character. Up to 1965 the Psychiatric Clinic was situated outside the city center; patients displaying mental disturbances were transferred to the psychiatric hospital. Since 1965 the number of consultations has grown considerably and at present it is the highest in the country. In 1973 a special full-time job was developed for a liaison psychiatrist which apart from clinical activities includes teaching and research work. Since 1968 the clinic has been kept standardized documentation of all consultations, with their results and conclusions periodically published. Due to this documentation the standard of consultations has noticeably improved. In many cases the consultant psychiatrist extended his activities to the patient's family, nursing staff, and also to a wider social environment of the patient [*Wardaszko-Lyskowska and Wlosinska,* 1976].

Despite this the organization and standard of consultations leave much to be desired. Thus, on the basis of a detailed analysis of consultations carried out by the Psychiatric Clinic of the Medical Academy in Warsaw, the following conclusions can be formulated: (1) Consultations treated as sporadic, time-limited actions do not fulfill their didactic function, nor do they fully expound psychiatric problems of psychosomatic patients. (2) Enormous scientific research potentialities are not utilized which appear in the situation where biological and psychosocial aspects of the problems converge. (3) For this reason the way consultations are conducted can satisfy neither the psychiatrists nor the physician. (4) In order to develop consultative psychiatry, consultant psychiatrists or clinical psychologists are gradually being employed in general hospitals, or consultation ambulatories set up. (5) The psychiatric clinic should be responsible for appointing a consultant psychiatrist who should maintain a close contact with it. This should enable the clinic to come closer to psychological-psychiatric problems of other departments of medicine. Moreover, this model bears upon the integration of the training of medical students, postgraduate, and specialization training [*Wardaszko-Lyskowska,* 1971b].

The Medical Academy in Poznan, where about 250 consultations are performed annually, can serve as another example. Uniform documentation of examinations renders possible comparative studies and constant improvement of this form of psychiatric work. Experiences gained allowed the following conclusions: patients in internal medicine units constituted half of all consultations; one third of these patients displayed functional and neurotic disturbances; about one quarter showed symptoms of apathy and lowered activeness in consequence of organic brain damage, while exogenous psychoses occupied a small percentage. In the majority of cases there were adequate grounds for consultations but only in 30% they were absolutely necessary [*Lisowska* et al., 1976].

Investigations into consultative psychiatry were carried out at the Psychiatric Clinic of the Medical Academy in Gdansk. On the basis of 4 years of psychiatric consultations in the Institute of Internal Diseases, psychotic complications in relation to various medical diseases were studied [*Januszkiewicz-Grabiasowa and Deptulski*, 1976]. Out of 632 consultations, complications of this type were found in 59 patients with pulmonary, circulatory, renal diseases, diabetes, acute pancreatitis, and other somatic diseases.

Apart from establishing therapeutic procedures – here the contribution of the consultant psychiatrist was vital – the above investigation may allow predictive criteria to identify individuals who become psychotic while undergoing medical treatment.

Investigations of *Borowski and Lukaszewicz* [1976] at the Medical Academy in Bialystok can serve as an example of the results of permanent psychiatric consultations in a university hospital. Consultations were mostly from internal diseases units as compared with surgical units. In the consulted patients psychogenic mental disturbances prevailed over the exogenous psychoses. Postsuicidal attempts constituted a large group.

The psychiatric ambulatory at the Central University Hospital of the Military Medical Academy in Lodz is an example of the way in which permanent consultations are organized. Psychiatrists and psychologists employed in both the ambulatory clinic and in the general hospital. Over a period of 3 years about 6,000 psychiatric examinations were performed including 604 consultations in various units of the hospital, most often neurological, internal diseases, surgical and ophthalmic units. Neurotic syndromes were most frequently diagnosed (50%), in the remaining cases psychoses or other psychopathological syndromes were found, as well as absence of mental disturbances.

During this period the number of patients visiting the ambulatory, as well as of psychiatric consultations increased by 100% as the result of improved understanding of emotional needs of patients hospitalized in somatic units of the hospital. Follow-up studies are disquieting since many patients examined by the consultant psychiatrist on somatic units (internal, surgical, gynecological-obstetrical, etc.) did not receive further psychiatric care. This group included the majority of patients with psychoses, and also patients after suicidal attempts [*Wysocka*, 1974]. Thus, to improve the effectiveness of psychiatric consultations the consultant psychiatrist should more fully participate in the work of the therapeutic team, the scope of activity of the psychiatric nurse and the social assistant should be extended, and clinical psychologist should be employed on somatic units as 'diagnostic liaison' between the team in charge of treatment and the consultant psychiatrist etc.

### Psychiatric Consultations in Provincial Hospitals

In those regions of the country where there are no psychiatric hospitals or where the distance to this hospital is considerable, a particularly important role belongs to the consultant psychiatrist, especially in the case of patients with a serious somatic illness, a postoperative state, traumas, poisoning, etc. One of the most difficult decisions which the consultant psychiatrist has to make is to leave these patients in the somatic unit and undertake treatment there, since their behavior may evoke not only anxiety and nervousness in other patients and staff, but also make treatment difficult or indeed impossible. Even in situations like this success can be achieved if the consultant psychiatrist can stimulate in the patient's environment and in the staff favorable attitudes, and apply effective treatment. For example, in the general hospital in the town of Chorzow, 25 patients in the internal diseases unit were successfully treated for acute psychotic disturbances [*Oczkowski* et al., 1976a, b]. It appeared that treatment in such conditions was not only possible but brought positive results equal to those that could be achieved in a psychiatric hospital, while medical treatment continued. Both the patients as well as their families were satisfied with the treatment on the somatic unit since the patients avoided a pejorative label of a psychiatric patient. These successful efforts induced a favorable change in the attitude of the whole staff of the hospital towards mental patients and enriched psychiatric knowledge of the other physicians.

In certain general hospitals consultations are performed by a psychiatrist employed in local mental health services, or by full-time, or part-time psychiatrist employed in hospitals who is not affiliated with a medical academy.

In the three hospitals in the town of Gdynia, in recent years 5 consultations have been performed per day, mostly in internal diseases, surgical, neurological and obstetrical-gynecological units. Most frequently mental disturbances diagnosed were organic brain damage, latent depressions, suicidal attempts, involutive depressions, reactive syndromes and others.

Many years of experience in Gdynia hospitals show that consultant psychiatrists are requisite for proper functioning of a general hospital and that opening full-time jobs of liaison psychiatrists in larger hospitals or complexes of hospitals is justified. The number of consulted patients supports the development of special psychosomatic and psychogeriatric units [Tyszkiewicz, 1976].

## Consultations in Various Disciplines of Medicine

The demand for consultant psychiatrists differs in various medical centers. Thus, for example, liaison psychiatrists are employed in several cardiosurgical centers, in transplantation centers, chronic dialysis centers, oncological units, in the case of the dying, etc. In recent years various investigations have developed in occupational and industrial medicine in which the roles of a psychiatrist and a psychologist are of equal rank to those of other specialists. In the Psychiatry Clinic in Krakow, investigations have been conducted for many years into the psychiatric aspects of vibration disease, chronic mercury poisoning and sulfur compounds poisoning [Szymusik, 1981].

Sporadically the consultant psychiatrist participates in investigations into the suitability for certain professions or work particularly hard, e.g. at high altitudes, or in situations of prolonged stress, etc. The range of psychiatric consultations has recently extended to various sport disciplines, especially record-seeking, e.g. boxing, climbing, parachute jumping, etc. The consultant has to decide whether the examinee is suited for the sports in question, estimate his personality predispositions, appraise his psychophysical fitness, and also estimate immediate and delayed consequence of practicing certain sports. The author of the present paper, for example, has for many years participated in the work of the Medical Commission of the Polish Alpine Club and the Volunteer Mountain Rescue Service investigating psychopathology of high mountain climbing, and delayed consequences of sojourn at high altitudes [Ryn, 1971, 1979a, b].

The consultant psychiatrist is particularly burdened with responsibility in the cases of attempted suicide. There are few areas where the consultant psychiatrist would so directly contribute to diminishing the mortality among patients not necessarily suffering from mental disturbances [*Domagalski*, 1976] as in suicidal attempts and there the preventive role of psychiatric consultations is most clearly reflected. In many toxicological units in Poland the psychiatrist is a permanent member of the therapeutic team. Sometimes a clinical psychologist is employed and then in every case he can request psychiatric help. The liaison psychiatrist effectively lessens the anxiety of the physician about the condition of the mental patient; he can also prevent unnecessary transfer of patients to psychiatric hospitals without real indications. He can intervene so that the patient can be directed to the outpatient department for further treatment or he can undertake various forms of psychotherapy to prevent another suicidal attempt [*Wiercioch*, 1976].

Children with mental disturbances are usually directed to children's mental health clinic or to the children psychiatric unit. In Poland, psychiatric consultations for hospitalized children in somatic units have been rare.

Patients undergoing treatment in the Institute of Mother and Child in Warsaw, and also in the Pediatric Institute of Medical Academies can remain under permanent care of children's psychiatrists. These medical centers have at their disposal either psychiatric consulting rooms for children where clinical psychologists are also employed, or have their own psychiatric units for children where – if necessary – children with mental disturbances can be transferred. Generally, a greater tolerance is observed of mentally disturbed children than of adult patients staying in somatic units. For this reason children, displaying mental disturbances during treatment in somatic units are less often consulted by the psychiatrist and more willingly treated in the original unit. For this reason it is worthwhile to report on the results of such consultations conducted in the children's unit of the Central University Hospital in Warsaw in the years 1973–1974. From among 3,200 children and young people treated during that period in the pediatric unit, 170 children were consulted by the children's psychiatrist. Mental disturbances were found in 83% of those examined, most frequently reactive neuroses, neuroses and behavioral disturbances. There was unfortunately very poor follow-up as to ambulatory care since only half of the patients reported to the outpatient department [*Osinska-Staniszewska and Komender*, 1976].

Old people, i.e. above 65 years of age, make up about 30% of patients hospitalized in Polish psychiatric hospitals. Close clinical evaluation of these patients reveals that many of them need not have been hospitalized.

Instead consultative psychiatric care would have been sufficient with concurrent and treatment by a general physician or internist. Since the 1970s,
the situation has been gradually improving. Many old patients who displayed only occasional psychotic disturbances remain in medical units yet
can take advantage of help from the consultant psychiatrist. Thus presence
of a psychiatrist within a general hospital induced other physicians to
modify their earlier prejudice towards mental patients.

The role of the consultant psychiatrist is difficult when a crisis develops
between treating physician and patient. A crisis like this may occur when
emotional ties between the patient and his physicians are formed, e.g. in
chronic dialysis units. This strong dependence arouses ambivalent feelings
that may express itself apparent through outbursts of aggression, resentment
and protest. One of the patients whom I consulted in the course of chronic
dialysis was a woman who was almost totally blind. She expressed her need
for contact with the environment and the need for being looked after via
screams, anger, outburst of temper, and even offensive verbal aggression
towards other patients and the staff. I was summoned for consultation repeatedly the dialysis staff tried to get me to transfer the patient to the psychiatric hospital to be brought back only for the dialysis. It seems that only
a psychiatrist, acquainted with the viewpoint of both sides could clearly see
the 'battle' being fought between the staff in the unit and the patient whose
basic psychic needs the staff could not satisfy. In this difficult problem it became my additional duty as a consultant to mediate between the two sides
in order to solve the conflict. Improvement was achieved after a number of
talks had been conducted directed at the physicians and other staff of the
unit which enabled them to solve their own emotional problems. The problems of dealing with such embottled units can be very stressful for the psychiatric consultant who could benefit from his own support systems.

Still different are the tasks of the Polish psychiatrist in medical commissions for invalidity and employment. As a rule, commissions like this do
not have a permanent psychiatrist. The most demanding task in this area is
the appraisal of the degree of invalidism for people with neurotic disturbances, and borderline cases. These problems usually go beyond the competence of general physicians and constitute a source of frequent diagnostic
errors in appraisal.

Psychiatric consultations in prison hospitals have a distinct character
resulting from an unusually difficult psychological situation (imprisonment,
danger of punishment, etc.), and psychopathological consequences of their
own kind. Psychiatric consultations in the units of hospital prisons are the

more important since the number of prison psychiatric units in Poland is insufficient and many prisoners with mental disturbances remain in general units.

Psychiatric consultations in the prison hospital in Szczecin can be described as a model solution. The forensic psychiatry unit of the Pomeranian Medical Academy in Szczecin is run by assistants of the Psychiatric Clinic of the Academy [*Rutkowski and Kramarz*, 1976].

Mental disturbances were found in one third of the patients. These were most frequently neurotic disturbances (mainly neurasthenic and hysterical), psychoorganic syndromes, endogenous and symptomatic psychoses, also reactive psychoses, personality disturbances, suicidal attempts and simulation of mental disturbances. Although this was basically a medical unit mental disturbances were the most frequent indication for hospitalization while somatic recommendations came next. Almost half of the patients should have been placed in a psychiatric or psychosomatic unit. Before permanent psychiatric consultative cooperation was undertaken, the patients remained in charge of physicians specialized in internal medicine who demonstrated attitudes of isolation and passively responded to the recommendations of the psychiatrist. In the results of the cooperation undertaken, part of the beds of the unit was assigned to mental patients and put in charge of physicians from the forensic psychiatry unit.

An insufficient number of psychiatric beds in prison hospitals necessitates hospitalization of part of the prisoners with mental disturbances in somatic units. The number of patients, type of mental disturbances, considerable diagnostic difficulties justify the conclusion that adequate care can only be delivered by full-time psychiatrists (liaison psychiatrists). It must not be forgotten, however, that this is merely a partial solution since the patients should in fact be placed in psychiatric units of prison hospitals.

### Difficulties and Perspectives

Crucial difficulties in the work of the consultant psychiatrist in Poland have been described by *Wardaszko-Lyskowska and Wlosinska* [1976]. Firstly, these are problems connected with deficiencies of the base and organization; secondly, problems connected with the psychological situation of the consultant; thirdly, problems caused by differences in outlook on the patient's problems and interests between the physician in charge of treatment and the consultant; and fourthly, difficulties connected with the tension in relations between the treated patient and the consultant. The consultant faces difficult problems, e.g. an excited patient in acute psychosis, a patient with dementive symptoms whose living conditions forbid discharging from the hospital and patients with complicated social-environmental problems when the family or people close to the patient try to take advantage of psychiatric consultations to place the patient in a psychiatric hospital. This happens most often in the case of patients with diagnosed alcoholism, drug addiction or personality disturbances, especially hysterical-impulsive with self-aggression, etc.

Experiences collected in everyday practice enable us to overcome the obstacles and methodically realize to an increasing degree, the educational function of consultations, as well as utilize them as the basis for research. It seems that despite the problems, consultative psychiatry within the Polish medical service system is undergoing a favorable evolution and reflects a general tendency towards integration.

Psychiatry should extend its participation in deciding upon the basic problems and conflicts of man in our times. In order to achieve this aim, psychiatrists should leave the confinement of psychiatric hospitals and consultation rooms and undertake a more direct and comprehensive dialogue, regardless of how difficult the task would be.

In the face of constant lack of psychiatrists, one of the ways to meet the enormous social need is consultative psychiatry. We can predict that in the future, psychiatry shall have to perfect and widen its special talents, and come much closer to other branches of medicine and nonmedical sciences which deal with psychophysical health of man. Training of psychotherapeutists, who could under the supervision of a psychiatrist conduct group psychotherapy, transactional analysis, or other forms of group therapy is yet another possible solution.

The necessity has arisen, therefore, for the language used in psychiatry to be purified of professional jargon in such a way that it can be understood by everyone thus becoming a suitable tool for discussion of universal problems of man and society.

*References*

Borowski, T.; Lukaszewicz, A.: Psychiatric consultations on the internal wards in the view of own observations (in Polish). Materialy XXXII Naukowego Zjazdu Psychiatrow Polskich, Szczecin 4–6 wrzesnia 1976. Polskie Towarzystwo Psychiatryczne, Warszawa-Szczecin 1976, pp. 14–19.

Domagalski, J.: Psychiatric consultations in acute intoxication wards (in Polish). Materialy XXXII Naukowego Zjazdu Psychiatrow Polskich, Szczecin 4–6 wrzesnia 1976. Polskie Towarzystwo Psychiatryczne, Warszawa-Szczecin 1976, pp. 26–28.

Falicki, Z.: Psychiatric problems in general hospitals (in Polish.) Psychiat. Polska *4:* 503–512 (1967).

Januszkiewicz-Grabiasowa, A.; Deptulski, T.: Psychosis with disorders of consciousness in internal diseases (in Polish). Materialy XXXII Naukowego Zjazdu Psychiatrow Polskich, Szczecin 4–6 wrzesnia 1976. Polskie Towarzystwo Psychiatryczne, Warszawa-Szczecin 1976, pp. 35–40.

Jaska, M.: The role of psychiatrist as consultant in the process of psychiatry integration made from experiences of nervous and mental disease hospital in Gniezno (in Polish). Materialy XXXII Naukowego Zjazdu Psychiatrow Polskich, Szczecin 4–6 wrzesnia 1976. Polskie Towarzystwo Psychiatryczne, Warszawa-Szczecin 1976, pp. 41–46.

Lipowski, Z.J.: Review of consultation psychiatry and psychosomatic medicine. I. General principles. Psychosom. Med. *29:* 153–171 (1967).

Lipowski, Z.J.: Review of consultation psychiatry and psychosomatic medicine. III. Theoretical issues. Psychosom. Med. *30:* 395–422 (1968).

Lipowski, Z.J.: Consultation liaison psychiatry in general hospital. Compreh. Psychiat. *12:* 461–465 (1971).

Lipowski, Z.J.: Consultation-liaison psychiatry: an overview. Am. J. Psychiat. *131:* 623–630 (1974).

Lisowska, J.; Rachowski, A.; Gasiorowska, B.; Kapelski, Z.: The analysis of the psychiatrist's participation in the diagnostic evaluation and treatment of the patients of other specialties (in Polish). Materialy XXXII Naukowego Zjazdu Psychiatrow Polskich, Szczecin 4–6 wrzesnia 1976. Polskie Towarzystwo Psychiatryczne, Warszawa-Szczecin 1976, pp. 65–74.

Lisowska, J.; Strzyzewski, W.: The role of consultant psychiatrist in certification of invalids (in Polish). Materialy XXXII Naukowego Zjazdu Psychiatrow Polskich, Szczecin 4–6 wrzesnia 1976. Polskie Towarzystwo Psychiatryczne, Warszawa-Szczecin 1976, pp. 60–64.

Oczkowski, Z.; Furman, J.; Makosz, K.: Treatment of acute psychotic disorders in non-psychiatric departments within the scheme of psychiatric consultation (in Polish). Materialy XXXII Naukowego Zjazdu Psychiatrow Polskich, Szczecin 4–6 wrzesnia 1976. Polskie Towarzystwo Psychiatryczne, Warszawa-Szczecin 1976a, pp. 104–108.

Oczkowski, Z.; Furman, J.; Makosz, K.: Expediency of psychiatric consultations in non-psychiatric departments (based on material collected in Chorzow) (in Polish). Materialy XXXII Naukowego Zjazdu Psychiatrow Polskich, Szczecin 4–6 wrzesnia 1976. Polskie Towarzystwo Psychiatryczne, Warszawa-Szczecin 1976b, pp. 100–103.

Osinska-Staniszewska, H.; Komender, J.: Psychiatric consultation on a pediatric ward (in Polish). Materialy XXXII Naukowego Zjazdu Psychiatrow Polskich, Szczecin 4–6 wrzesnia 1976. Polskie Towarzystwo Psychiatryczne, Warszawa-Szczecin 1976, pp. 109–114.

Piotrowski, A.: Psychiatry and the psychiatrist in general hospitals (in Polish). Zdrow. publ. *83:* 137–141 (1972).

Piotrowski, A.; Szemis, A.; Wysocka, A.: Mental patients in general medical care (in Polish). Biul. Inst. Psychoneurol. *4:* 56–67 (1978).

Rutkowski, R.; Kramarz, E.: Specific of psychiatry consultation in the conditions of a prison hospital (in Polish). Materialy XXXII Naukowego Zjazdu Psychiatrow Polskich, Szczecin 4–6 wrzesnia 1976. Polskie Towarzystwo Psychiatryczne, War- szawa-Szczecin 1976, pp. 115–120.

Ryn, Z.: Psychopathology in alpinism. Acta med. polona *3:* 455–469 (1971).

Ryn, Z.: Motivation and personality in high mountain climbing. Can. alp. J. *62:* 57–58 (1979a).

Ryn, Z.: Nervous system and altitude. Syndrome of high altitude asthenia. Acta med. pol. *2:* 155–169 (1979b).

Schrammowa, H.: Analysis of 1,044 psychiatric consultations in Poznan clinics and hos- pitals in the years 1954–1959 (in Polish). Przegl. Lek. *7:* 210–215 (1960).

Szymusik, A.: Mental health in industry (in Polish). VI Konferencja Naukowa Psychia- trow Polskich i Czechoslowackich, 7–9 IX 1980, Lodz-Plock. Pamietnik. Polskie Towarzystwo Psychiatryczne, Lodz, 1981, pp. 147–152.

Tyszkiewicz, M.: Psychiatric consultation – a bridge between a general hospital and the psychiatric health service (in Polish). Materialy XXXII Naukowego Zjazdu Psy- chiatrow Polskich, Szczecin 4–6 wrzesnia 1976. Polskie Towarzystwo Psychiatryczne, Warszawa-Szczecin 1976, pp. 131–135.

Wardaszko-Lyskowska, H.: Psychiatric consultations in general hospital (in Polish). Psychiat. Polska *5:* 525–531 (1971a).

Wardaszko-Lyskowska, H.: Some problems of consultation psychiatry (in Polish). Psychiat. Polska *4:* 475–480 (1971b).

Wardaszko-Lyskowska, H.; Lukaszewska, H.; Szyszkowski, W.: Psychiatric consultation in various departments of the Medical Academy in Warsaw (in Polish). Psychiat. Polska *5:* 136–145 (1971).

Wardaszko-Lyskowska, H.; Wlosinska, I.: Analysis of the difficulties in realization of the clinical, educational and scientific goals of the psychiatric consultations (in Polish). Materialy XXXII Naukowego Zjazdu Psychiatrow Polskich, Szczecin 4–6 wrzesnia 1976. Polskie Towarzystwo Psychiatryczne, Warszawa-Szczecin 1976, pp. 146–150.

Wiercioch, L.R.: Children's poisoning suicide attempts and psychiatric consultations (in Polish). Materialy XXXII Naukowego Zjazdu Psychiatrow Polskich, Szczecin 4–6 wrzesnia 1976. Polskie Towarzystwo Psychiatryczne, Warszawa-Szczecin 1976, 151–155.

Wilczkowski, E.: Necessity of the construction of a psychiatric clinic of the medical academy in the University General Hospital (in Polish). Neurol. Neurochirur. Psych. Pol. *2:* 381–385 (1952).

Wlosinska, I.; Frindt-Zajaczkowska, A.: Psychiatric consultations of the patients with chronic renal insufficiency treated with chronic dialysis and transplantation (in Polish). Materialy XXXII Naukowego Zjazdu Psychiatrow Polskich, Szczecin 4–6 wrzesnia 1976. Polskie Towarzystwo Psychiatryczne, Warszawa-Szczecin 1976, pp. 160–166.

Wysocka, A.: Psychiatric consultations on the somatic wards (in Polish). Psychiat. Polska *5:* 515–522 (1974).

Z. Ryn, MD, Associate Professor of Psychiatry, Department of Psychiatry, Medical Academy, ul. Skarbowa 4, PL-31-121 Kraków (Poland)

Adv. psychosom. Med., vol. 11, pp. 88–108 (Karger, Basel 1983)

# Consultation-Liaison Psychiatry in Israel

*Jacob Avni*

Psychiatric Unit, Hadassah University Hospitals, Jerusalem, Israel

## *Historical Perspectives*

Until the mid-nineteenth century, the standards of public health in Palestine were very poor. Limited medical help was offered mainly by the Christian missions. When the first wave of Zionist immigration to Palestine occurred (1843–1881), seven physicians arrived and the first Jewish hospital was opened here. From the beginning of the 20th century more and more physicians came to Palestine with the immigration waves. The Labor Sick Fund (Kupat-Holim) and the American Hadassah Organization began to develop health services in Palestine before the First World War: hospitals, outpatient clinics, mother and child health centers, school health services, and nursing schools. The pioneers of modern medicine were physicians from Eastern Europe; but in the thirties a mass of Jewish doctors escaping from Germany and Austria arrived, bringing with them the latest developments in medicine. After the establishment of the state in 1948 medical needs were suddenly increased by the huge waves of immigration. The new Ministry of Health with the help of existing services coped successfully with many severe problems. In accordance with the Zionist immigration policy, every doctor from any medical school abroad is licensed to work in Israel. This has a negative influence on the level of medical services, mainly in the outpatient clinics of the Labor Sick Fund which serve the ambulatory medical needs of 80% of the population. The four medical schools produce well-trained physicians whose medical education is similar to the American model.

The physician-patient ratio in Israel is approximately 2.1 per 1,000 population, one of the highest in the world. There are 135 hospitals. The number of general hospital beds per 1,000 population at the end of 1980 was

2.95. 93% of the population have medical insurance. The hospitals belong to the government and to the Labor Sick Fund or the municipalities. There are almost no private general hospitals. The central hospitals are teaching medical centers and have intensive care units, neurosurgery and open heart surgery departments. They are well-equipped and deliver good medical care. Private practice is rare and very few doctors work independently. There are numerous outpatient clinics all over the country but their physicians are rather isolated from the hospitals. More than 850 mother and child health centers do excellent work in this field of public health. In the last decade emphasis has been laid on developing and improving the field of family practice.

### Mental Health Services in Israel

#### General Psychiatry

The history of mental health services in Israel follows the development of the general medical services in the country, however always lagging behind it. The first psychiatric institute in Palestine was established in Jerusalem under the Turkish rule in 1902. It was founded by a Jewish charity society called Ezrath-Nashim in order to nurse and maintain the mentally ill. In the period of the British mandate during the twenties, two other mental institutions were added – in Bethlehem and in Bnei-Brak. Subsequently some small private 'pensions' were opened to solve the problem of mental hospitalization for the quickly growing population in the Holy Land. In 1942, the first modern mental hospital, Gehah, was opened by the Labor Sick Fund with 70 beds. Bethlehem mental hospital served mainly the Arab population. Soon, after the establishment of the state of Israel in 1948, masses of Jewish survivors of the holocaust in Europe and immigrants from Arab countries arrived in Israel. The needs for public psychiatric care changed rapidly. This brought about the opening of eight public psychiatric hospitals during a relatively short period. The ratio of psychiatric beds today in Israel is 2.1 per 1,000 population. Future plans are to have 2.8 beds per 1,000 population divided as follows: 1 per 1,000 in acute hospitals; 1 per 1,000 in work villages; 0.6 per 1,000 in custodial nursing homes; 0.1 per 1,000 in general hospitals, and 0.1 per 1,000 in special institutions. Today Israel has 40 psychiatric hospitals: eleven belong to the government; three to the Labor Sick Fund; two to public societies, and the rest are private. There are also three work villages and two psychiatric hostels. In the United States the rate of psychiatric inpatients per 100,000 population shrank by more than 40% between 1950 and 1970. In Israel this rate did not change significantly between 1965 (2.58 per 1,000) and 1970 (2.68 per 1,000). Up until 1979 there was a moderate decrease to 2.28 per 1,000, despite the fact that the outpatient services increased by more than double during this period. The explanation of these facts is debatable [19].

The first psychiatric outpatient clinics were part of the psychiatric hospitals and isolated from outpatient clinics of other medical specialties. These clinics dealt mainly with severe psychiatric disturbances. The preventive attitude in psychiatry and the focusing on mental hygiene were much developed by psychologists and psychiatrists of the Youth-Aliyah – the Zionist organization that dealt with the welfare of children and adolescents amongst the immigrants. The experience of immigration and wars and the phenomenon of the Kibbutz partially moved the emphasis in the mental health field in Israel towards community psychiatry and preventive mental health programs. This direction was expressed by the establishment of mother and child clinics, municipal school psychological services and consultation services to general practitioners and paramedical personnel. The number of psychiatric outpatient clinics in Israel is now 83 and only 20 of them belong to hospitals. Israel is divided into 23 areas each served by specific mental health agencies. Ambulatory psychiatric treatment and hospitalization is free of charge to all the population. This includes the psychiatric hostels, day centers, and ten centers for treating drug addicts and alcoholics. The overall psychotherapeutic orientation is psychodynamic, influenced by the Isracli Institute of Psychoanalysis. In the mental health centers crisis intervention and short-term therapies are practiced in addition to long-term individual and family therapy. The psychobiological approach and the latest developments in the psychopharmacological field are applied in all the psychiatric facilities where necessary. Behavioristic methods and other therapeutic modalities are comparatively rarely used.

### Psychiatric Departments in General Hospitals in Israel

The formation of psychiatric consultation services and the opening of psychiatric wards in general hospitals were important steps in the development of modern psychiatry in Israel. These steps were strongly influenced by the ideas of psychosomatic medicine that arrived from the United States after the end of the Second World War. In addition, the War of Independence and the massive immigration that followed were directly responsible for the integration of psychiatry into the general hospitals.

In 1948, some months after the establishment of the state of Israel, *Gerald Caplan* opened a psychiatric ward in the military hospital in Haifa. It consisted of 20 beds and dealt mainly with war neuroses. In the same year, *Caplan* opened in addition a psychiatric ward in the general civil hospital, Rambam, in Haifa. These were the first psychiatric departments in general hospitals in Israel. The civil department hosted mainly refugees from the holocaust in Europe or immigrants from Arab countries. Active treatment included electroconvulsive therapy, narcoanalysis and continuous narcosis. Individual and group psychotherapeutic sessions were introduced. Teaching of psychiatric nurses, social workers and clinical psychologists took place in the general hospitals. The consultations to the wards were begun as strictly patient-centered consultation.

In 1951 a 30-bed Psychosomatic Department was opened by *Julius Zellermayer* in Tel Hashomer Hospital, near Tel Aviv, a military and civilian hospital of approximately 650 beds. The department was needed mainly in order to deal with psychosomatic and psychiatric disorders in young soldiers. In 1954 a small psychiatric ward was opened by *Milton Rosenbaum* as part of the university hospital of Hadassah in Jerusalem. It consisted of ten beds only and the emphasis was on psychosomatic aspects of psychiatry and consultation service for other departments. Today, there are in Israel psychiatric departments in eight out of 38 general hospitals. The other hospitals have psychiatric consultation provided by psychiatric hospitals or clinics or by individual psychiatrists.

## The Department of Psychiatry in Hadassah Medical Center

### History of the Department

Hadassah hospital in Jerusalem was the first university hospital in Palestine and has been since its establishment in 1939 the leading medical center of the country. The department of psychiatry in Hadassah was the first one to exist in a teaching hospital in Israel. Relating the history of this department and the personal history of some of the pioneer psychiatrists involved would aid in understanding the origins and circumstances of the development of general-hospital psychiatry in Israel.

*Friedrich S. Rotschild* was born in Germany and completed his medical studies in Munich. He became an assistant of *Kurt Goldstein* and *Frieda Fromm-Reichmann* and was a neuropsychiatric consultant in the university hospital in Frankfurt. In 1933 he was fired with all the other Jewish doctors in Germany. In 1936 he escaped to Jerusalem. *Rotschild* was accepted to the local psychoanalytic society but his main persistent interest has been to correlate and integrate the knowledge in neurology, psychiatry, medicine and philosophy. In his special way *Rotschild* has been a psychosomaticist although remote from the main theoretical streams of psychosomatic medicine in the thirties. In 1948 he was asked by the head of neurology to become the psychiatric consultant of Hadassah. One of his first tasks was to deal with war neuroses of soldiers and citizens of Jerusalem which suffered greatly in the War of Independence. He worked individually with his patients, using some short tests for assessment of the patient's personality, including special neurological tests, habitual postural positioning and graphology. For treatment he used short psychotherapy of one to three sessions, sometimes hypnosis or the Schultz autogenous training.

*Milton Rosenbaum* was born in Cincinnati, Ohio, but always had a very special interest in Jerusalem. In 1954 he was already one of the well-known figures in the field of psychiatry and psychosomatic medicine in the United States. *Rosenbaum* contributed to the understanding of the dynamics of many of the psychosomatic disorders. He had a strong interest in the role of psychiatry in general medicine, the patient-physician relationship, and the role of the psychiatric department in a general hospital. As a result he was invited by the Hadassah Hebrew University Medical School to establish and head a department of psychiatry in the existing general hospital. This department was started in July 1954. The unit was an open one and consisted of ten beds situated in the courtyard of the hospital. The main emphasis was on psychosomatic aspects of psychiatry, and consultation service for other departments. Some of the pillars of the medical school resented the new American fashion of a psychiatric department in the general hospital. To a large extent it was the good personal relationship of *Rosenbaum* with many physicians and teachers in the medical school that helped to overcome gradually and partially the suspicion and resentment. Weekly psychosomatic case presentations were begun in the Department of Medicine for all the staff and students. Weekly psychosomatic conferences took place in the psychiatric ward. Regular conferences were held later with the Department of Pediatrics and the Department of Family Medicine. While being psychoanalytically oriented, the medical orientation of the department was emphasized from the beginning in its regime.

In 1955 *James Mann*, who was at that time teaching psychiatry in Boston University Medical School, was invited to replace *Milton Rosenbaum* who returned to the United States. *Mann* was already a distinguished figure in the Boston Institute of Psychoanalysis. In Jerusalem he invested most of his time in teaching and supervising the residents, psychologists, social workers and psychiatric nurses. *Mann* taught dynamic psychotherapy in its different forms applied to the outpatient clinic, the psychiatric ward and to psychiatric consultation. Gradually more people in the hospital began to accept the idea of a psychiatric ward there, although for some others the name of psychiatry was still a shameful stigma.

*Julius Zellermayer* was in the thirties a young neuropsychiatrist in the General University Hospital of Vienna. Vienna was the center of struggle between different theories and thoughts – mainly between the Kraepelinian view in psychiatry and Freudian psychoanalytic theory. *Schilder, Hartmann, Stengel* and *Korsakoff* were some of the names who opened new directions and thoughts in psychiatry. The ideas about psychosomatic and somato-psychic processes began to find support even in the conservative institution of Viennese medicine. In 1938 Hitler's troops marched into Austria. *Zellermayer* escaped immediately to Tel Aviv. In 1942 he was called to serve as a psychiatric consultant in Tel Hashomer hospital near Tel Aviv. His concern was to diagnose and treat psychosomatic conditions in the Department of Internal Medicine. In 1951 he was appointed the head of a new psycho-somatic department in Tel Hashomer hospital. A few years later *Milton Rosenbaum* invited *Zellermayer* to come to Jerusalem and head the young Department of Psychiatry he had founded there. *Zellermayer* began to head the department in 1956. The department also included Prof. *Rotschild* and two residents. Another psychiatrist came from Yale, New Haven, in 1956 and brought with him a psychosocial orientation. The chief clinical psychologist came in the same year bringing Roger's client-oriented approach. Above all, the department remained psychosomatically and psychoanalytically oriented. The different approaches were integrated slowly into an eclectic attitude.

In 1958 *J.J. Groen* from Holland was appointed head of one of the two Internal Medicine Departments in Hadassah hospital. *Groen* was by that time one of the well-known names in the field of psychosomatic medicine. Soon after his coming to Hadassah a cooperative venture was founded which consisted of regular common seminars and rounds and the formation of 'Balint groups' in the hospital. Later on there was even interchange of residents between the two departments for a period of 6 months. Nevertheless the coming years saw the great hopes for fruitful cooperation unfulfilled. In 1961 a new university medical campus was erected in Ein-Karem, near Jerusalem. The physical integration of the psychiatric ward on the eighth floor of the new hospital raised anxieties and opposition in some heads of other departments. Fortunately, the management of Hadassah was understanding and supportive. A small ward of 16 beds was opened side by side with Surgery, Gynecology and the other specialties. In 1967 the ward was increased to 30 beds.

In the new medical center at Ein-Karem a busy psychiatric outpatient clinic began to function, serving the community and providing consultation services to the other outpatient clinics in the hospital. This clinic has been the only one in Jerusalem specializing in psychosomatic medicine.

### Structure of the Department

The Psychiatric Department of Hadassah is divided into the ward, the outpatient clinic and the consultation service units of the Ein-Karem and Mount-Scopus hospitals. The adult outpatient clinic has about 7,000 visits per year and the pediatric psychiatry clinic 6,000. Physicians, psychologists and social workers form the staff. Referrals are mostly from other clinics in town. The ward is semiopen and has at present 20 beds fully occupied. The average patient's stay is 45 days. Some of the patients are primarily psychotics or severe neurotics who also have some physical pathology. Some others have psychiatric problems secondary to a physical ailment. Other patients are called 'psychosomatic' when psychosocial aspects play an important role in their physical disease. Such patients may be treated in the medical or in the psychiatric ward depending on the psycho-vs.-somatic balance and the motivation of the staff and patient. In the ward there is a therapeutic milieu. Two senior psychiatrists and three residents, two psychologists and two half-time social workers together with psychiatric nurses, a physiotherapist and occupational therapist comprise the staff on the ward.

### Psychiatric Consultation-Liaison Services in Hadassah

Hadassah Medical Center in Ein-Karem, Jerusalem, has 700 beds. This is the biggest hospital in Jerusalem and accepts patients from all over the country. It has all the basic and highly specialized departments including intensive care units and open-heart surgery. The other teaching hospital of Hadassah is on Mount-Scopus. It includes the basic departments, intensive care units and the Department of Rehabilitation. It has 300 beds and functions mainly as a regional hospital for the eastern part of Jerusalem. No positions are allocated specifically for consultations. One senior psychiatrist is in charge of consultation services in each hospital. The other four seniors and four juniors are attached to consultee departments. The juniors begin their consultative work in their second year of residency under supervision of the seniors. Three seniors are trained psychoanalysts and the other two are psychodynamically oriented; however, the psychiatric practice in consultation, as in the ward and clinics, is suited to the individual patient. Emphasis is placed on understanding the actual stresses and traumas, their personal meaning for the patient and his ways of coping with the situation. Patients are enabled and encouraged to speak for the purpose of obtaining information, ventilation and abreaction. The psychiatrist is supportive in attitude. Many times he supplies the patient with important information about his illness in an optimistic-realistic spirit. Psychopharmacological drugs are used in more than half of the cases. Most frequently used are minor tranquilizers, followed by anti-psychotics and antidepressant drugs, in this order. When psychotherapy takes place it is reality and goal-oriented along the lines of 'medical psychotherapy' described by *Kimball* [12]. In some rare cases hypnosis or behavioristic techniques are used.

Referrals for psychiatric consultation come from the physicians in the wards via a special form. In many cases the initiative comes from the nurse or social worker of the department concerned; but even then she has to convince the physician to call the consultant. Most of the referrals relate to symptoms of depression, anxiety or behavior that disturbs the staff or other patients. Confusion, insomnia and lack of organic diagnosis are other common reasons for requesting consultation. Occasionally the consultant is requested to assess patients whose physical disease seems to be affected by situational psychosocial factors. Many of these patients have 'classical' psychosomatic diseases like hypertension, duodenal ulcer or bronchial asthma; but other conditions like hematological, autoimmune or infectious diseases are included in this group. As long as these patients stay in their original wards, the psychotherapeutic investment of the consultant is generally secondary and additional to the organic therapy. Only in relatively few cases where the psychological aspect is clearly dominant is the patient, with his consent, transferred to the psychiatric ward where he is treated mainly by psychiatrists (or psychologists) with the cooperation of the 'physical' consultant of the ward. Patients who threaten suicide or display behavior intolerable to the staff are also transferred.

Departments can not be divided into those who have positive or negative attitudes toward the psychiatric service. It seems that the consultation relationship depends mainly on the motivation and abilities of the psychiatric consultant and on his acceptance by the consultees. Even the classical distinction between the accepting medical departments and the rejecting surgical departments is not valid in our experience. Successful liaison connections existed for long periods in Plastic Surgery, the Orthopedic Department and in the Dialysis Unit. Departments which are considered now to be rejecting had a good psychiatric liaison service in the past when some consultant was especially interested in them. A study was done in Hadassah hospital [9] in an attempt to reveal the attitudes of the consultee physicians toward the psychiatric consultation service. The main findings were that the physicians found the psychiatric consultation helpful. Many of them want regular participation of the psychiatrist in the routine of their departments and in case conferences. The findings indicate that the expectations of the departments of surgery were mainly for a consultation service while those of medicine were for a liaison service. The author suggests that 'emotional problems of the consultants, i.e. ambivalence about their profession is the source of the common tension between psychiatric consultants and other physicians'.

A short survey of consultative psychiatry and liaison medicine in Hadassah Hospitals' departments may demonstrate the wide variety of interrelationships between psychiatry and other specialties.

Consultative psychiatry is referred to when a psychiatrist comes to the consultee department solely when requested, from outside this department and from outside its specialty. He gives his opinion or advice, but he himself is not a part of the process of decision making. Liaison medicine is referred to when the psychiatrist is accepted as part of the consultee department. In this case he has adequate knowledge in the field of this department and he takes part in the process of decision making concerning the patient.

*The Internal Medicine Departments* have always been the main consumer of psychiatric consultations. Each of the departments requests 25–30 consultations per month. In some of the cases there are several contacts with the patient as well as with the nurse, physician or family. Occasionally the consultant takes part in staff meetings and discussions about the patient. The four departments of medicine are somewhat different regarding their attitude to psychiatry; but all of them recognize the importance of psychological factors in many of their patients, although they have doubts about the practical aspects of this knowledge.

Psychiatric activities in the departments of medicine can be considered as semi-liaison, and stable in nature.

*The Departments of Surgery* have different relationships with psychiatry. Both parties are critical about the psychiatric consultation service and both are unfortunately correct. Requests for the psychiatrist are mainly for urgent and severe problems. Surgeons are often not available to speak to before or after the consultation. Hospitalization periods are generally short, the surgeons are mostly surgery oriented and body oriented. Initiatives for psychiatric consultations come too often from the nurses. Conditions in the surgical wards are not favorable for interviewing the patient and recommendations by the consultant to the team are often not fulfilled. The disappointed psychiatrists tend to limit their interventions in the surgical cases to the most necessary matters. This often brings the surgeons to feel that psychiatric consultations do not add much to the management of their patient. Nevertheless it must be said that some surgeons are sensitive and understanding to the psychological aspects of their patients. Thus they prevent much of the patient's anxieties and depression and render our consultation less often needed.

With the *Department of Plastic Surgery*, a very good psychiatric liaison has been existing for many years. The psychiatrist concerned had a special interest in the psychological aspects of burns, cosmetic surgery and pain and made himself an integral part of the department. Participating regularly in surgical rounds and staff meetings became a rule. Emotional problems of the families and of the team have been dealt with as part of his investment. A good peacetime working relationship enabled a quick transfer to a suitable wartime cooperation [1] which was not possible in other surgical departments [6]. *The Department of Orthopedics* had in the past a 2-year period of successful psychiatric liaison whilst one of the psychiatrists had a genuine interest in this department and its special problems. Soon after his leaving the department the framework built with toil disintegrated to minimal unsatisfying psychiatric consultation.

*The Rehabilitation Department* has a very special character. In the past this department had good psychiatric liaison service, mainly following the wars. After the Six-Day War of 1967, the Ministry of Defence found it necessary to establish a post for a psychiatrist in this department, mainly to aid in the rehabilitation of soldiers with spinal cord injuries. Some years later there were misunderstandings and frictions between the psychiatric consultants and the Department of Rehabilitation. In 1977 the department was transferred to Mount-Scopus and extended to two wards comprising 40 beds. Since then two half-time psychologists serve in cooperation with the psychiatrist in a psychiatric liaison. This includes participation in all rounds, staff meetings and case conferences.

*The Dialysis Unit* was started in Hadassah in 1966 and almost from the beginning a psychiatrist was asked to participate intensively in its work.

Her first tasks were to help in selecting the most suitable patients by predicting compliance, suicidal tendencies, etc. The staff of the unit was under continuous extreme stress and welcomed any aid. The psychiatrist was interested in medicine and willing to learn as much as possible about dialysis. These conditions favored the existence of a successful psychiatric liaison in the Dialysis Unit. The psychiatrist examined all patients prior to dialysis and participated in the selection-rejection decisions. She undertook psychotherapy for patients during dialysis and participated in all staff conferences. Later on fruitful research was begun with the cooperation of a psychologist and the nephrologist.

*The Oncology Department* has a half-time psychologist who has been trained in this specific area. In cooperation with the psychiatric consultant variable clinical work is done. This includes individual consultations and therapeutic sessions with patients and families. Psychopharmacological treatment is used not only for anxiety, depression or psychotic reactions but also for intractable pain syndromes and nausea. Hypnotic sessions are also used to alleviate anxiety, pain or nausea. Group therapy for postmastectomy women has been existent for the past 2 years.

*Other departments* like Neurology, Dermatology, Neurosurgery, Hematology and Urology all use psychiatric services in the form of consultations.

*Emergency rooms* in both hospitals have 70,000 visits per year and provide much emergency psychiatric material. The psychiatric residents are on duty around the clock and a senior is at their disposal for consultation. They are called to see patients who attempted suicide or who suffer from acute anxiety, intoxication, delirium, etc. Here the resident has to differentiate psychiatric from organic pathology or to identify the psychiatric aspects of complex medical or surgical situations. Conditions in emergency rooms are hardly suitable for a psychiatric interview and demands to have a separate psychiatric emergency room were not fulfilled for years. The emergency rooms also serve the army in the Jerusalem area, and this enables the service to deal with military psychiatry.

*Intensive care units*, surgical and coronary, exist in both hospitals. Psychiatric consultations are generally requested only for cases of acute psychoses, severe anxiety or depression and suicidal attempts. No psychiatrist has ever become an integral part of these closed societies. It is possible that they would have accepted more help if an experienced psychiatrist had shown more interest in the units. At present only in severe emotional crises do the nurses appeal for help; and with the cooperation of the units' physicians, sessions are arranged to deal with the extreme tensions and anxieties that arise in such units. The dehumanized atmosphere of the units appears to repel the psychiatrists although it should attract their initiative and investment.

*The Department of Child Psychiatry* in Hadassah was opened in July 1977 under the chairmanship of *Gerald Caplan* with four senior child psychiatrists and three residents assisting him. In some ways this department was a continuation of the Lasker Mental Hygiene and Child Guidance Center of Hadassah founded by *Caplan* in 1949. The new Department of Child Psychiatry began to offer consultation services to the child patient population in other departments, including also their families and staff. A high proportion of consultation work was invested in 90 beds in Alyn Orthopedic Hospital for Children. Special links were formed between the Department of Child Psychiatry and the Departments of Pediatric Surgery and of Pediatrics. Children with burns, major congenital anomalies or undergoing surgical treatment of external genitalia were screened routinely. Good working relationships were formed with the ward social worker, nurses and physicians. In the Pediatric Departments, a similar process has been taking place. *Caplan* et al. [4] describe four patterns of child psychiatrist cooperation with other departments: the autonomous psychiatric unit, consultation, collaboration and executive partnership. These represent a gradient of increasing participation of psychiatrists inside the other departments in the treatment of patients, in case responsibility and in administrative authority over the service system. The executive partnership is often called a psychosomatic unit. In Hadassah such a unit has recently been established, with subunits inside each pediatric department of the two hospitals.

### Psychiatric Consultation Services in Israel

#### Special Problems in the Patient Population

The most important of these are immigration, the holocaust, the wars and terrorism. One of the special features of Israel is that it was established for the purpose of the ingathering of Jewish exiles. Within 30 years the number of its citizens increased from 600,000 to about four million; and this happened mostly by mass immigration. The immigrant to Israel, as to any country, loses many external supportive frameworks. The confidence he previously derived from familiarity with the surrounding way of life and identifications with family, neighborhood, work and ethnic groups, gives way to anxieties and insecurity. The strange language and cultural habits, the new manners and values, the uncertainty as to housing, work, and political status, and often the separation from family and friends, all increase the strain. Interethnic frictions and tensions add a further load to the pressures against which they must stand firm [3, 17]. The acute psychological problems of the new immigrant are manifested by increased general anxiety, insecurity and regression, with increased needs for dependence. People may develop irritability and aggressiveness, withdrawal states, paranoid reactions or traumatic neuroses. These reactions are seen in each new wave of immigration, while the recent immigrants gradually become old-timers and, for most of them, the psychological reactions are reduced. Some never adapt to the new surroundings, while in many others adaptation is partial and superficial. When these people are physically ill and hospitalized, their problems of belonging and migration are reemphasized. In psychiatric consultation in Israel the psychiatrist must be multilingual in order to do his work well. The main problem, however, is not the language, because most people acquire the Hebrew language quickly, but the differences in cultural backgrounds. To this is added the existence of ethnic minorities in Israel: Moslem Arabs, Christian Arabs, Druze and some other small groups. A psychiatric consultant has to know much about tradition, beliefs and prejudices, moral codes and accepted ways of expressing feelings in order not to do damage. He has to know even more in order to be helpful. Yemenite Jews may have signs of small burns, specially made at home to heal all kinds of ailments. Arab families will ask to take the dying patient home to die there decently. A very religious Jewish married woman is not allowed to stay alone with a male consultant in a closed room, but if the door is even symbolically open, then it is kosher. Jews from Europe and America distinguish readily between physical and psychological problems, while Jews from Arab countries, like Arabs themselves, tend to express their feelings through bodily complaints. Worries, anxieties and depression are often expressed by complaints of fatigue and general or circumscribed pains. Nevertheless, only after learning and understanding the varied cultures and traditions, one can see that deeply similar processes and defence mechanisms are active under dissimilar masks.

A very special phenomenon, prevalent mainly in Israel, is the psychological syndrome of Nazi holocaust survivors. These victims who went through hell in Europe have lasting chronic psychopathological symptomatology which has been described by some authors [13, 17, 18]. They suffer from different expressions of anxiety, sleeping difficulties and mnestic disturbances. Other changes are manifested as low frustration tolerance and aggressive outbursts. Permanent difficulties in socialization and affectively relating to other people have been described. Survival guilt feelings and paranoid attitudes are common. In recent years more and more specific psychopathology of the second generation of concentration camp survivors has been described. When holocaust survivors become sick and are hospitalized their anxieties are often worse than those of others. The dehumanization experience of hospitalization often causes resurrection of the old trauma. Their clothes are taken away, they are given striped pajamas and put with strangers into a big hall. They lose their independence identity and privacy and are separated from their loved ones. It is quite common for these anxieties to be manifested clinically, sometimes as exaggerated fears of the medical or surgical procedures, but frequently as nightmares with memories of the concentration camp. In the case of psychotic breakdowns occurring in intensive care units, the delusions and hallucinations of concentration camp survivors have their content taken from the experience of the holocaust. For some of the holocaust survivors each war or terrorist act is a cause for reexacerbation of their anxiety.

The five wars between Israel and the Arab countries made great demands on the consultation services all over the country. The small teams of psychiatrists in general hospitals, especially in surgical wards, were increased by volunteer psychiatrists, clinical psychologists, social workers and laymen. The leaders of these teams were the consultants that had worked in the surgical departments in peacetime. Almost every war was different from the others in weapons used and the character of the resulting injuries. In the Six-Day War and the period following it, the psychiatric consultation services had to deal with head and spinal-cord injuries, while in the Yom Kippur War many burns from tank fights filled the burn units. Rehabilitation of amputees, paraplegics and the burned is one of the important tasks of psychiatric consultation services.

In surgical wards the consultants are generally psychiatrists only. In rehabilitation wards and centers, psychologists do most of the consultative work, many times as part of the team of these wards. In peacetime between the wars, there are many cases of 'civil' catastrophes when bombs are placed by Arab terrorists in supermarkets or bus stations causing death and injuries. Consultation services are trained to deal with the acute psychological reactions of the patients and their families. Much psychiatric work is invested in trying to avoid posttraumatic reactions in these patients. Psychiatric consultants in the general hospital train first aid and civil defence workers in how to deal with the injured, the families and the gathering crowd from the point of view of psychiatric prevention and treatment.

### Consultation Activities

The psychiatric activities within the Hadassah hospitals have been described in detail in order to exemplify the character of similar activities in other teaching hospitals. Four psychiatric wards exist in university hospitals and another four belong to peripheral hospitals that do not teach medical students. These hospitals treat mainly the rural population, while most of the patients of the academic hospitals come from the big cities. The eight departments have only 224 beds altogether, each one having between 17 and 45 beds. Some of the hospitals have small psychiatric day-care units. Most of the other general hospitals obtain consultation services from adjacent psychiatric hospitals or clinics. The small private hospitals have their own arrangements with private psychiatrists who are called mainly for severe cases.

### Status

Psychiatry in Israel has a relatively low status in comparison with internal medicine and surgery. It attracts a low proportion of our medical graduates as a vocational choice. It is considered mostly as a 'minor' subject in the medical schools, although almost half of the hospital beds in the country are psychiatric. The public's attitude in Israel toward psychiatric problems and patients is often one of fear and shame. The physicians often share this attitude. Many of them are relatively free from prejudices in this matter; but many others hesitate even to ask their patients if they have had psychiatric problems or treatment in the past. This is one reason why psychiatry entered the general hospital only after the bitter War of Independence. The physicians in these general hospital departments represent psychiatry in medicine although they are different from most other psychiatrists. They have more interest and knowledge in specialties other than psychiatry, and are generally closer to the medical model than to the model of the social sciences. They are more reality oriented, problem oriented and time oriented than their colleagues in the mental hospitals. While these psychiatrists are hardly accepted as equals by physicians of other professions, they are viewed with ambivalent feelings by other psychiatrists. Some encouragement to the brave representatives of the profession, but also suspicion and envy, are directed towards this group of psychiatrists. The government and Labor Sick Fund psychiatric services do very little to increase the number of psychiatric wards or beds in the general hospital. The Israeli Psychiatric

Association is not understanding enough with regard to the interests of the psychiatric wards in general hospitals; and they are discriminated in the area of residency programs. Among the other psychiatrists as well as among the physicians of the other specialties in the general hospitals, the psychiatric consultants are considered to be hybrids and strangers. Psychiatry is merely tolerated in most hospitals. In most cases consultation is requested only for severe symptoms or problems. Liaison medicine is often claimed by psychiatrists to exist but is rare as a real long-standing phenomenon. The wars were an important factor in forming liaison frameworks. In such times of existential dangers it is almost impossible to deny the psychological needs of wounded soldiers, their families and staff. Examples of this model were the Departments of Plastic Surgery (Burn Units) in Beer Sheva and Jerusalem during the Yom Kippur War [1, 21] and the organization of Hadassah and Beilinson Hospitals during that war [6, 16]. These liaison organizations were temporary and disintegrated after some months, not only due to budget shortages, but also to a lack of motivation from both sides.

Liaison in peacetime exists in some departments where the consultee and consultant have a strong motivation for it. This may be a research interest, as in the case of the dialysis unit, gynecology and obstetrics or rehabilitation in our hospitals. The question of budget is important in the difficult economic situation of Israel. Research money goes more to special fields like dialysis, open heart surgery or oncology. These units have also more liaison services than the others.

In the sixties the big interest in psychosomatic medicine gave the psychiatric consultant an important status in medicine, almost equal to the status of the internist himself, in relation to some patients. With the years the concept of 'psychosomatic' has been extended from certain specific diseases to include aspects of almost all health disorders. Gradually, disappointment with the time-consuming nature of psychotherapy, conditional on the availability of experts, together with the development of new drugs (for UD, hypertension etc.) devalued the emphasis on psychosomatic aspects in physical disease.

*Teaching*

The Hadassah-Hebrew University Medical School was inaugurated in 1949 and is the first and largest of the four existing medical schools in Israel. The other three are in Tel Aviv, Haifa and Beer Sheva. The duration of the course is 6 years. The 1st year is premedical, the next 2 preclinical and the last 3 are clinical years. 1 year of rotation internship is mandatory. The total number of graduates per year in Israel is under 300. Psychiatry is generally considered a 'minor' subject; and this is well reflected in the attitudes of the schools and members of the faculties. Only in Beer Sheva is psychiatry being taken more seriously and thought of as part of the behavioral sciences.

Frontal lectures in psychology and psychiatry have been going on for years with disappointing results. As in the other medical professions, the important teaching is done in the clinical years as bedside teaching in small groups. 5th-year medical students come to our ward in groups of six for a period of 6 weeks of clinical clearkship. One of these is dedicated to child psychiatry. Other medical students go for a similar period to one of three affiliated psychiatric hospitals in Jerusalem or to the psychiatric ward that exists in Kaplan General Hospital in Rehovot. During the preclinical years very little is taught about medical psychology and psychosomatic medicine. In the clinical years, some of the students are exposed to general hospital psychiatry in the emergency room and in the framework of our consultation services. The students accompany the consultants when possible and thus bedside teaching can be accomplished. During the past years an additional means to teach medical psychology has been employed. When students enter the different departments, we give them seminars on the psychiatric aspects of surgery, gynecology, etc. More emphasis should be put on this teaching framework because of the relative importance of medical psychology in the future experience of all our students. These seminars outside the Psychiatric Department give reality to the unity of body-mind for the student and also the importance of psychology and psychiatry as part of the medical practice.

Students of psychology and of social work have their clinical experience mainly within the psychiatric ward and outpatient clinic, but not in the consultation service. Social workers are placed in certain departments. They take care of the social problems of the patients but are often also involved in helping them with psychological situational reactions. In many cases they accept guidance or even supervision from the psychiatrist involved. Nurses are frequently the best source of information for the psychiatrist; and in some departments the consultant invests in them by teaching principles of medical psychology applied to nursing. In some cases group meetings of social workers, nurses and residents of the same department have been conducted.

Supervision of residents who practice consultation in the hospital departments is most important; but unfortunately, this method of teaching is not always properly practiced due to the pressure of time and circumstances. Other frameworks for teaching include presentations at clinical conferences

for the whole hospital and discussions at case conferences with the staff of
the host departments. Special courses are given to groups of general physicians from the outpatient clinics of the Labor Sick Fund. These are group
discussions on subjects of medical psychology in the general hospital and
also in the practice of outpatient clinics, mainly surgery, medicine, gynecology and obstetrics. We participate constantly in courses given to the civil
defence forces and senior students concerning handling multiple traumas
and reactions to mass civil disasters in war and peace. Residency training is
5 years, as in most specialties in medicine. It does not include an obligatory
period in psychiatric consultation service or in a psychiatric ward in a
general hospital. Nevertheless, 6 months' training in consultation is recognized as part of the period necessary for specialization. Board examinations in psychiatry were introduced in Israel some years ago and the people
involved in medical psychology try to make this material an obligatory part
of the curriculum and examinations.

### Research

Research is the least developed aspect of psychiatry in Israel [10]. This
has probably to do with the fact that psychiatry lagged behind the progress
of medicine in Israel for many years. Until recent years most of the psychiatric hospitals were far from the influence of medical schools. During
the past years more psychiatrists have been showing interest in research,
mainly in psychopharmacology.

Of the departments of psychiatry in general hospitals, some do no
research at all because of the pressure to give clinical services and the lack
of sufficient personnel. Some research is done in the teaching hospitals
where 'publish or perish' is the law. Articles published in the field of consultation psychiatry and liaison medicine can be divided into different groups.
Some are case reports about psychosomatic, somatopsychic or neuro-
psychiatric cases. These appear in English in international journals, and
sometimes in Hebrew in local journals. There are also papers about the
subject of psychiatric consultation and liaison where the authors summarize
their services and experiences in their hospital. These papers relate to a
specific experience like consultation in the emergency room [7], pediatric
service [4] or the department of gynecology and obstetrics [5]. Other papers
describe an experience which was unique like consultation or liaison during
the wars [1, 16, 21]. Some of the psychiatrists working in the field of medical
psychology have written chapters in books dedicated to this field [2, 11, 20]
and some books on psychosomatic and somatopsychic issues have been

published [8]. Systematic and fruitful research developed mainly where a liaison organization existed like in the Dialysis Unit in Hadassah. Such research is encouraged by the liaison framework and also improves and strengthens the bond of the psychiatrist and the consultee department. We have cited merely a few examples of research done in the field of consultation-liaison psychiatry in Israel.

The impression is that this research is developing slowly and its future depends on the prospects of this field in Israel.

### Conclusions

The advancement of psychiatry in Israel has lagged behind that of general medicine. Not withstanding its important achievements psychiatry's status is more similar to the situation in England [15] than to what is happening in the United States [14]. It is still rejected and feared by the public, including physicians, and discriminated by government and public health services. It is relatively unattractive to medical graduates. The relatively severe problems of mental health in Israel are not reflected in the share which psychiatry receives in medical teaching, budgets or research. The history and present state of general hospital psychiatry in Israel reflects the mutually ambivalent relationships between psychiatry and general medicine. Psychiatric consultation and liaison services were founded mainly as a result of severe situational needs and against strong opposition. There is not enough understanding for, or future planning in this medical branch. Psychiatric departments exist in only eight out of 38 general hospitals and often have to face suspicion, hostility or discrimination from both frontiers of general psychiatry and general medicine. Under the difficult economic conditions they are the first ones to be threatened and constricted by rivals and sharks. Nevertheless, the existing services reflect important lasting achievements in the process of the integration of medicine and psychiatry in this country. Psychiatric consultation-liaison services represent the refined new concept of psychosomatic medicine. The unity of body-mind is a truth which has daily new proofs in both fields of research and therapy. This is the real strength of general hospital psychiatry. It is not a hybrid but an important step toward the real thing – the reunification of medicine into a comprehensive theory and method of treating the whole human being. This is why in Israel, like in many other countries, psychiatric consultation and liaison medicine will endure, progress and spread in the hospitals and from them to all the community health services. Despite all the doubts about past investments in this field, more and more efforts should be directed to teaching, research and service so that past errors may be corrected and future ones prevented.

## References

1 Avni, J.: Psychiatric care of burn patients during wartime. Psychother. Psychosom. *26:* 203 (1975).
2 Avni, J.: The severe burns. Adv. psychosom. Med., vol. 10, p. 57 (Karger, Basel 1980).
3 Caplan, G.: Mental hygiene contributions to the resettlement of immigrants in Israel. Ment. Hyg., Concord *36:* 607 (1952).
4 Caplan, G. et al.: Patterns of cooperation of child psychiatry with other departments in hospital. J. Prevention (in press, 1982).
5 Hertz, D.G.: Problems and challenges of consultation psychiatry in gynecology and obstetrics. Psychother. Psychosom. *23:* 67 (1974).
6 Hertz, D.; Kaplan De-Nour, A.: Effects of war on psychiatry in a university hospital. Psychiat. Opinion (May 1975).
7 Hes, J.: Stress and challenge of the emergency room of the general hospital. Psychiatria clin. *9:* 112 (1976).
8 Kaplan De-Nour, A.; Czaczkes, J.W.: Chronic hemodialysis as a way of life (Brunner/Mazel, New York 1978).
9 Kaplan De-Nour, A.: Attitudes of physicians in a general hospital towards psychiatric consultation service. Ment. Hlth Soc. *5:* 215 (1978).
10 Kaplan De-Nour, A.: Israel; in Usdin, World studies in psychiatry, vol. 3 (4), p. 1 (1979).
11 Kaplan De-Nour, A.: Dialysis center. Adv. psychosom. Med., vol. 10, p. 132 (Karger, Basel 1980).
12 Kimball, C.P.: Medical psychotherapy. Psychother. Psychosom. *25:* 193 (1975).
13 Klein, H.: Survival and revival; psychodynamic studies of holocaust survivors and their families (Yale University Press, New Haven (in press, 1982).
14 Lipowski, Z.J.: Holistic-medical foundations of American psychiatry: a bicentennial. Am. J. Psychiat. *138:* 888 (1981).
15 Lloyd, G.G.: Liaison psychiatry from a British perspective. Gen. Hosp. Psychiat. *2:* 46 (1980).
16 Maoz, B. et al.: Psychiatry in a general hospital in wartime. Kupat Holim Yb. *4:* 143 (1975).
17 Miller, L. (ed.): Mental health in rapid social change (Jerusalem Academic Press, Jerusalem 1972).
18 Musaph, H.: The second generation of war victims: psychopathological problems. Israel J. Psychiat. Relat. Sci. *18:* 3 (1981).
19 Rahav, M.; Popper, M.: Trends in the delivery of psychiatric services in Israel in the years 1965–1979. Unit of Information and Evaluation, Mental Health Services, Ministry of Health (1980).

20 Rosenbaum, M.; Hertz, D.G.: Gastrointestinal disorders; in Wittkower, Warnes, The psychosomatic approach to medical practice (Harper & Row Medical Department, Maryland 1977).
21 Solnit, A.J.; Priel, B.: Scared and scarred – psychological aspects in the treatment of soldiers with burns. Israel Ann. Psychiat. *13:* 213 (1975).

Jacob Avni, MD, Senior Lecturer in Psychiatry, Hadassah University Hospitals, P.O. Box 24035, Jerusalem (Israel)

Adv. psychosom. Med., vol. 11, pp. 109–126 (Karger, Basel 1983)

# Consultation-Liaison Psychiatry in the United Kingdom

*Dennis Gath, Richard Mayou*

University Department of Psychiatry, Warneford Hospital, Oxford, England

## *Historical Development of Psychiatry in the General Hospital*

Before the Second World War almost all British psychiatrists worked in large mental hospitals, providing largely custodial care for severely disturbed involuntary patients. There were only two university departments, the Maudsley Hospital and the Edinburgh department. There was little private practice. The few out-patient clinics, which were mainly concerned with neurotic problems, were mostly in London teaching hospitals and were staffed by doctors who thought of themselves as specialists in psychological medicine. The only general hospitals in Britain to have psychiatric beds were Guy's Hospital and the Middlesex Hospital which had six beds each.

In 1948 the start of the National Health Service brought a single system encompassing the different types of hospital – voluntary and municipal, general and psychiatric. Almost all psychiatrists became full-time salaried employees of the Health Service, whilst only a minority had any part-time private practice. The country was divided into administrative regions, and this made it possible to plan comprehensive psychiatric services for each local area. The main priorities were to improve the care of the chronically disabled in large institutions and to develop the out-patient and community treatment of mental illness.

The Ministry of Health put forward an ambitious Hospital Plan (1962), in which the development of general hospital psychiatry was prominent. The aim was to close the large asylums and replace them by small units in district general hospitals. In retrospect, this radical plan can be seen as over-ambitious and underfunded. The traditional mental hospitals have remained but with fewer beds. Nonetheless considerably more psychiatrists have been based in district general hospitals providing services to a defined catchment area.

Alongside this development of district general hospitals, the teaching hospitals began to expand their psychiatric units. By the late 1960s university departments of psychiatry had been established in almost all medical schools. As they had no responsibility for catchment areas, their medical staff had the time and opportunity for teaching, for treating acute and neurotic problems and for providing consultation-liaison on medical wards. In recent years, however, the responsibility for a local community has been taken on increasingly by teaching hospitals as well as by district general hospitals.

Despite differences in working conditions, academic psychiatrists and those working in mental hospitals have shared a similar pragmatic and eclectic outlook, with little or no adherence to psychoanalysis. This approach has reflected the dominant influence of the Maudsley Hospital on training, and the demands of heavy clinical responsibilities on a small specialty. Since 1971, this broad approach has been further encouraged by the founding of the Royal College of Psychiatrists, which has helped to unify the profession and to supervise and improve training throughout the country.

This history of eclectic psychiatry mainly practised outside the general hospitals meant that the traditional psychosomatic medicine of the 1930–1960 period had little impact upon British clinical practice. There were no close links between the main academic centre, the Maudsley Hospital, and any general hospitals. Only a few psychiatrists in general teaching hospitals had any opportunity to see medical and surgical patients, to teach or do research. Hence present-day general hospital psychiatrists have inherited few developed theories about the relationship between physical and psychological illness.

*Consultation-Liaison Psychiatry*

After 1948 the increasing numbers of psychiatrists in general hospitals began to see more and more patients referred by physicians and surgeons. In several teaching hospitals special services were provided in which one or more experienced psychiatrists provided consultation that was rapidly available. In the early 1960s several accounts were published of such services and their referral patterns [*Fleminger and Mallett*, 1962; *Kenyon and Rutter*,

1963]. The main reasons for referral were requests for diagnostic advice, for management of acute psychiatric disturbance, and for assessment of deliberate self-harm. In the 1950s this last group made up only 10–20% of consultations, but were regarded as particularly in need of psychiatric assessment. In 1961 a Ministry of Health circular recommended that all deliberate self-harm patients admitted to hospital should be assessed by a psychiatrist before discharge. The subsequent large rise in such admissions has put increasingly heavy demands on psychiatric consultation services.

Whilst the need for consultation in general hospitals has been widely accepted, there has been relatively little interest in liaison psychiatry in its narrow sense, i.e. that of a psychiatrist as a full-time member of the medical team. Individual psychiatrists have made notable contributions and in the sixties some university departments attached senior staff to medical teams. *MacLeod and Walton* [1969] described joint case conferences and teaching in the academic medical unit in Edinburgh. The academic unit at the Middlesex Hospital, which was established in 1961, made liaison psychiatry one of its main priorities, emulating the Rochester model of Engel and Romano [*Crisp*, 1968]. However, experiments of this kind were not common.

### Current State of Consultation and Liaison

#### Clinical
Although the Royal College of Psychiatrists has specialist groups for subjects such as forensic psychiatry and psychotherapy, there is no such group for consultation-liaison psychiatry, which has no national forum. It is therefore difficult to form a picture of current practice. However, it is clear that only a small minority of psychiatrists in Britain have a special interest in consultation-liaison, and less than ten consultants have a full-time interest. Most general hospital consultation is undertaken by general psychiatrists. Probably all general hospitals have some form of psychiatric service, almost always providing emergency consultation rather than personal liaison. Published statistics tend to come from the more energetic departments but they still indicate lower referral rates than in the United States. Most referrals are for deliberate self-harm and it is in the assessment of this problem that the main advances have been made. For example, there have been several promising developments in the multidisciplinary management of deliberate self-harm.

The trend has been for psychiatrists to develop close links with particular medical units rather than to establish full-time liaison. Apart from the assessment of deliberate self-harm, there has been little attempt to develop multidisciplinary teams in medical and social wards. The traditional discipline of medical social work has remained detached. Clinical psychology is so far a small discipline largely confined to working with specialist psychiatry; less than 50 psychologists work in general hospitals, mostly in departments of neurology and rehabilitation.

A detailed picture of current clinical practice is provided by a survey of the 20 psychiatric administrative areas in Scotland [*Brooks and Walton*, 1981]. Although Scotland is not typical in having only six general hospital psychiatric units, the overall picture is probably representative of Britain as a whole. In 1979 few areas had psychiatrists with a special interest or responsibility for consultation or liaison. Referrals were usually made impersonally on request forms, and drug overdose was the commonest reason. The authors' overall impression was of unsatisfactory communication between psychiatrists and other hospital doctors before and after referral. In most areas there was a wish to improve and expand liaison services, but lack of resources was a major obstacle.

In Great Britain, consultation-liaison services are undoubtedly less elaborate than in the United States, with the exception of services for deliberate self-harm, which have been extensively developed. The main reasons for this are shortage of psychiatrists, and the priority given by the National Health Service to the treatment of psychiatric disorder referred directly to the psychiatric services. When *Russell* [1973] examined the working week of typical British psychiatrists, he found that no time was available for consultation in the general hospital. Other possible reasons include the lack of a psychosomatic tradition, and the resistance of physicians and surgeons to psychiatric referral [*Mezey and Kellet*, 1971].

It is possible that in Britain, where the general practitioner is responsible for primary psychiatric management, fewer psychiatric problems are admitted to medical and surgical beds. Hospital physicians and surgeons may also take the view that psychological problems should be assessed by the patient's general practitioner before referral to a psychiatrist.

### Teaching Medical Students

In the fifties and sixties psychiatry was gradually accepted as an essential part of the teaching of clinical medical students. This was encouraged by the influential Royal Commission on Medical Education and by the national bodies responsible for educational funding (University Grants Commission) and for medical curricula and examinations (General Medical Council). Apart from the teaching of specialist psychiatry, most medical schools have attempted to teach psychological aspects of general medicine and surgery. The most popular approach has been lectures and seminars, whilst ward round teaching by liaison psychiatrists has been less common. In some medical schools there are also limited opportunities for students to be attached to consultation units during their period of psychiatry training.

In 1981 a working party including the Association of University Teachers of Psychiatry [1982] surveyed medical schools to enquire about teaching of consultation-liaison psychiatry for medical students. Of the 25 British medical schools, 21 responded and their replies provide the best available information about the state of teaching and indeed of consultation psychiatry in Britain.

Three medical schools had a specialist in consultation-liaison psychiatry, 17 had at least one general psychiatrist with a special interest, but two had neither. In three schools there was no consultation-liaison teaching; of the remaining 22, half provided teaching during student attachments to medical firms, whilst the other half provided teaching during attachments to specialist psychiatry. It appeared that almost half the medical schools provide no practical experience of consultation-liaison psychiatry apart from the assessment of self-poisoning.

### Training Psychiatrists

Trainee psychiatrists (registrars) usually take part in 3-year rotational training schemes in preparation for their higher qualification in psychiatry (Membership of the Royal College of Psychiatrists). Training is regulated by the Royal College, which has recommended that trainees should have experience of consultation-liaison psychiatry.

The AUTP obtained information on registrar training from the organisers of rotational training schemes. It appeared that most registrars have some experience of the assessment of deliberate self-harm, two thirds of working in a general hospital, and half of seeing patients referred from medical and surgical wards. 29% of the schemes had at least one rotating consultation-liaison post, whilst 25% had registrar posts with links with medical or surgical units.

Trainees who have passed the examination for Membership of the Royal College of Psychiatrists become senior registrars for a further 3–4 years, before applying for permanent consultant posts. Senior registrar training is regulated by the Joint Committee on Higher Psychiatric Training,

and this too has recommended that trainees should have experience of consultation-liaison psychiatry. However, the Joint Committee's impression is
that few training schemes have posts providing substantial experience in
consultation-liaison psychiatry.

### Research

In Britain the main research interest has been deliberate self-harm.
Since the early survey by *Stengel* [1964] there has been extensive research on
the epidemiology of both completed suicide and deliberate self-harm. Psychological and social determinants of suicidal behaviour have been identified, together with factors influencing the risk of repetition of such behaviour.
Recently there has been increasing interest in evaluating various methods
of intervention for suicidal behaviour.

Research has also shown high prevalences of psychiatric disorder
amongst medical out-patients [*Shepherd* et al., 1960] and medical in-patients
[*Maguire* et al., 1974]. Such studies have been greatly helped by the introduction of standardised methods of identifying psychiatric morbidity, such
as the General Health Questionnaire [*Goldberg*, 1972], Standard Psychiatric
Interview [*Goldberg* et al., 1970] and the Present State Examination [*Wing*
et al. 1974].

A third research interest has been the description and measurement of
the psychological sequelae of different medical or surgical illnesses and
procedures. These studies have also made increasing use of standardised
measures of mental state. The range of current interests is illustrated by the
published proceedings of a recent conference in London [Society for Psychosomatic Research, 1981].

### Future of Consultation-Liaison Psychiatry

It is widely agreed amongst British psychiatrists that effective consultation services are required for the assessment and treatment of the psychological problems that are so common in medical and surgical practice. There
is less agreement about the best ways of organising such services in the
future [*Lloyd*, 1980; Editorial *British Medical Journal*, 1981]. It seems unlikely
that consultation-liaison psychiatry will become a separate subspecialty but
increasing numbers of general psychiatrists will probably take an interest in
it. Consultation-liaison psychiatry is also likely to gain strength because
many psychiatrists regard it as valuable in the education of trainee psy-

chiatrists and clinical medical students. On the other hand, liaison psychiatry in the narrow sense (the psychiatrist as a full-time member of the medical team) is unlikely to take root in Great Britain. This is because there is a shortage of psychiatrists and of resources within the National Health Service, and because priority continues to be given to improving psychiatric hospitals and psychiatric care in the community.

## Consultation-Liaison Psychiatry in Oxford

For the population of 510,000 living in the City of Oxford and surrounding areas, psychiatric services are provided mainly by two psychiatric hospitals, one of which houses the University Department of Psychiatry. Together these form a Sector of Psychiatry, which is autonomous and administratively separate from medicine and surgery. Treatment is available without selection to anyone living in the catchment area. Patients are admitted under the provisions of the National Health Service, and do not pay for their treatment. They are drawn from all socio-economic classes, and are representative of the background population.

Since 1979, consultation-liaison services in Oxford have been largely provided by a unit in the John Radcliffe Hospital, which is the main teaching hospital of several in the City. The unit is part of the University Department of Psychiatry and has good modern accommodation for consulting, teaching and secretarial work. There are no in-patient beds, but these are available at one of the psychiatric hospitals about 1 mile away. In addition to this service, other psychiatrists within the Sector provide consultation in several areas of specialist medicine, including paediatrics, geriatrics, physical rehabilitation, and the care of the dying.

The senior staff of the consultation-liaison unit is led by a full-time National Health Service Consultant Psychiatrist (Dr. E.B.O. Smith), who has overall charge of the unit, and two members of the University Department of Psychiatry who each attend for several sessions a week. The junior medical staff consists of one or two trainee psychiatrists (registrars), who spend 6 months full-time in the unit as part of their 3-year training, and a number of higher trainees (senior registrars) who each attend one afternoon a week in rotation to supervise junior staff. The latter rather piecemeal arrangement is the best that can be managed with available resources.

The psychiatric orientation of the medical staff is the same as in virtually all teaching hospitals in the United Kingdom, that is, eclectic and not

adhering to any single doctrine or specialised style of practice. Psychodynamic principles are sometimes used but not more than others; for example, behavioural principles are widely used as well. The non-medical
staff includes psychiatrically trained nurses and a social worker. The unit
has three main kinds of activity: (i) providing a clinical service to two types
of patient: (a) those who have attempted self-poisoning or self-injury (sometimes called attempted suicide or parasuicide), (b) those with medical and
surgical conditions; (ii) educating and training junior doctors, clinical medical students and nurses, and (iii) research. Each of these activities will be
reviewed in turn.

## Providing a Clinical Service

The service has largely been developed by the Clinical Director, Dr.
E.B.O. Smith and is mainly consultative. There is less emphasis on liaison
in the narrow sense, that is, psychiatrists belonging to medical teams.

### Management of Deliberate Self-Harm
In the past decade, there has been a steady rise in the numbers of patients referred after deliberate self-harm or self-poisoning. The numbers of
referrals now average 800–900 a year.
In the early seventies a service was set up in which nurses and social
workers carry out most of the assessment and treatment of such patients,
under supervision from psychiatrists. This was a new development in the
United Kingdom, and it is only one of several models adopted in this
country. The service was established to provide assessment and treatment
for patients with the minimum delay. Clinical research had shown that most
of the patients were not psychiatrically ill, but rather facing distressing personal and social problems that they could not solve. It therefore seemed a
good idea that nurses and social workers should participate in both assessment and treatment.
An important principle is that thorough training must be provided for
non-medical staff who take on this role. This is provided in several ways;
for example, manuals are provided explaining principles of assessment and
treatment; seminars are given on suicidal behaviour and related topics such
as depression; interviewing techniques are demonstrated with live and tape-
recorded interviews, and trainees' interviews are tape-recorded for discussion
with supervisors. All staff are trained to carry out a systematic interview

which aims not only to estimate suicidal risk reliably, but also to evaluate the full range of problems facing individual patients and the possible ways of tackling them. Relatives and friends are interviewed whenever possible.

In clinical practice, nurses and social workers are given full medical support. Each afternoon a 'senior cover meeting' is held, at which a higher psychiatric trainee (senior registrar) and the emergency team review current patients. Assessments of new patients are discussed and treatment plans agreed in a multidisciplinary setting.

Treatment in the unit is offered to 45–50% of patients assessed. The others are mainly discharged to the care of the general practitioner, or referred to a psychiatric hospital as out-patients or in-patients. For most patients, treatment can be provided by nurses and social workers; the few patients who are psychiatrically ill are allocated to one of the team's psychiatrists [*Hawton* et al., 1979].

Treatment consists mainly of brief counselling focussed on current problems. This is usually provided on a flexible out-patient basis by the member of staff who made the assessment. Occasionally patients are visited in their own homes. Day care is available, as is group therapy for selected patients. Up to one third of the patients are offered access to the service through a direct telephone line.

Several evaluative studies suggest that this kind of service works well. Nurses and social workers assess over two thirds of referrals to the unit. It has been shown that this has resulted in much more rapid assessment and in a lower occupancy of much-needed medical beds. It has also been demonstrated that the trained non-medical staff can carry out assessments of suicidal behaviour as reliably as psychiatrists [*Catalan* et al., 1980], and that the patients are well satisfied.

### Consultation Service to Medical and Surgical Firms

A consultation service is provided chiefly to the four main medical units in the John Radcliffe Hospital, each of which receives general medical patients and also has a special medical interest. Each is staffed by consultant physicians and by physicians in training. For two of these firms consultation is provided by the National Health Service Consultant Psychiatrist and by one psychiatric registrar; for the other two firms it is provided by two senior members of the University Department of Psychiatry and by one registrar. This division of duties means that psychiatrists and physicians can form closer working relationships. The psychiatrists attend medical case conferences, but their role is essentially in consultation rather than liaison.

In addition to this linkage with the medical firms, consultation is also provided on a less formal basis to the surgical firms, to the Casualty Department, and to physicians and surgeons in the other general hospitals in the Oxford teaching group.

Referrals are usually dealt with on the day they are received. The first assessment is made by the registrar, who interviews the patient and discusses the problem with the ward staff. The registrar then discusses the patient with the consultant psychiatrist. Advice to the physicians, or any appropriate psychiatric treatment, is provided by the registrar with guidance from the consultant.

### Liaison Service

In a few medical subspecialties a psychiatric service of the liaison type is provided. This means that the psychiatrist collaborates with the physicians in the management of all the patients, not just those referred to him because of suspected psychiatric disorders. This kind of service is provided in the units for renal dialysis and transplant, rehabilitation of the physically handicapped, and care of the dying.

## Education and Training

Teaching and training in consultation-liaison psychiatry are provided for junior doctors, clinical medical students, and nurses.

### Junior Doctors

Education and training are provided to junior trainee psychiatrists (registrars) in the Oxford area in several ways. First, they can attend two academic courses which are held 1 day a week during university terms at one of the psychiatric hospitals. These courses provide 72 hours of seminar teaching on the sciences basic to psychiatry, and 144 hours on clinical psychiatry. During the first year of the clinical course, there are six seminars on general hospital psychiatry, covering topics such as: an introduction to psychosomatic medicine; physiological and biological factors in psychosomatic illness; psychiatric aspects of physical illness. During the second year, there are six further seminars covering topics such as: the sick role and illness behaviour; psychiatry in the general hospital; psychological aspects of surgery; psychological aspects of dying; psychological aspects of pain.

In addition to this academic teaching, most registrars obtain in-service experience in the general hospital psychiatric unit. This is a 6-month full-time attachment that involves mainly consultation-liaison work, and also some assessment and treatment of deliberate self-harm. Two or three times a week throughout the attachment, registrars attend ward rounds concerned with both teaching and management of patients. Seminar teaching is also provided in the general hospital psychiatric unit, covering such topics as: the concept of psychosomatic medicine; dying and bereavement; self-poisoning and self-harm; hysteria; psychiatric aspects of epilepsy.

Apart from trainee psychiatrists, general practitioner trainees take part in their own 3-year vocational training course in the Oxford hospitals. Most of them work for 3 or 4 months in the general hospital psychiatric unit, where they take part in consultation-liaison work, assessment and treatment of self-poisoning patients, and emergency duties. They also attend the academic seminars in the unit.

### Clinical Medical Students

On completion of their pre-clinical training in medical sciences, Oxford medical students take a clinical course lasting 2 years and 9 months. In the first clinical year, they have an 11-week full-time attachment to a medical firm at the John Radcliffe Hospital, during which they have a weekly seminar with a senior psychiatrist. This seminar teaching is closely related to clinical problems presented by the medical in-patients known to the students. The aim is to cover most or all of the following topics: skills of interviewing; anxiety states and depressive illness; atypical depression; organic mental states; hysteria; alcoholism; psychosexual problems; suicide and deliberate self-harm; psychotropic medication; eating disorder; pain; malignant disease; dying and bereavement; psychiatric disorder after surgery; management of acutely disturbed patients.

During their second clinical year, clinical students have an 8-week full-time attachment to the department of psychiatry. This provides apprentice-type experience and some seminar and tutorial teaching. Most of them work in one of the two psychiatric hospitals, but a few work in the general hospital psychiatric unit, where they participate in the assessment and treatment of patients in the consultation-liaison service and in the service for attempted suicide patients. All the students attend a seminar on the management of deliberate self-harm.

In the last few months of their clinical training, students have a second 11-week attachment to a medical firm. Here again weekly seminars are provided by psychiatrists. This time the course is concerned more with revision and with discussion of practical psychiatric problems that are likely to arise in the forthcoming year as a house officer (intern).

Psychiatric Research in the General Hospital

Psychiatric research in the general hospital has not adopted the traditional psychosomatic themes that were largely concerned with psychodynamic factors in the aetiology of physical illnesses such as bronchial asthma, peptic ulcer and ulcerative colitis. Instead it has examined the psychological impact on patients of various medical conditions and procedures, and of the factors influencing their outcome. Research in Oxford has been largely concerned with developing research methods suitable for this kind of enquiry. Emphasis is laid on the use of standardised methods for defining, detecting and measuring psychiatric morbidity. This has involved the use of established screening questionnaires such as the General Health Questionnaire [*Goldberg*, 1972] and measures of mental state, such as the Standardised Psychiatric Interview [*Goldberg* et al., 1970] or the Present State Examination [*Wing* et al., 1974]. In addition, workers in Oxford have developed a self-administered scale for measuring social functioning [*Cooper* et al., 1982b], and various structured schedules for measuring sexual adjustment, menstrual functioning, and psychological and social recovery after physical illness.

Emphasis has also been placed on using prospective research designs whenever possible, particularly in examining questions for which earlier retrospective studies gave inconclusive results. For example, baseline psychological and social measures are taken before surgical procedures and the same measures repeated at intervals afterwards. This avoids retrospective distortion which is likely to occur when patients are assessed only after the event. Finally there has been emphasis on studying patient samples that are not only of adequate size for statistical analysis, but also as homogeneous as possible and representative of a defined population.

*Psychiatric Studies of General Medical Conditions*

Three examples will be given to illustrate the range of research on general medical conditions.

*Psychiatric Morbidity and Referral in the General Medical Wards.* In this study psychiatric morbidity amongst 230 medical in-patients was detected by a two-stage screening procedure using the General Health Questionnaire and the Standardised Psychiatric Interview [*Maguire* et al., 1974]. Of these patients, 23% were judged to be psychiatrically ill, the commonest diagnosis being depressive illness. 12% (27) of the patients were referred to a psychiatrist. Whilst referral was releated to severity of psychiatric illness and to previous psychiatric illness, the main determinant appeared to be the degree to which psychiatric illness was obtrusive or created problems in management. Half the patients who were psychiatrically ill were not detected as such by the ward staff.

In a second study, this group of medical in-patients was followed up later [*Hawron*, 1981]. It was found that in many cases, the psychiatric disorder detected previously persisted during an 18-month follow-up. A number of patients with poor psychiatric outcome had not been referred to a psychiatrist at the time of the original admission. The presence of psychiatric disorder at the original admission was associated with an increased mortality rate.

*Psychosocial Aspects of Myocardial Infarction.* In a prospective study of patients suffering from myocardial infarction, psychological and social outcome was assessed at 2 months and 1 year later. Considerable morbidity was found in patients and their families [*Mayou*, 1979]. A subsequent project has developed reliable measures of social adjustment for physically ill patients [to be published]. These are now being used in a prospective investigation of the psychological and social consequences of coronary artery surgery.

A recent study evaluated two forms of cardiac rehabilitation, exercise and counselling, which have been regarded as valuable in improving psychological, medical and social outcome after infarction. Although exercise training appeared to improve confidence during the early stages of convalescence, it appeared to be of little benefit to cardiac function, everyday life and emotional state. This suggested that some accepted beliefs about the value of rehabilitation may be unfounded, and may result from the biases of uncontrolled studies [*Mayou* et al., 1981].

*Psychiatric Studies of Patients in Terminal Care.* An intensive study was made of the types of problems presented by 49 patients referred to a psychiatrist in a terminal care unit. It was concluded that a psychiatrist can play a useful role in such a unit, particularly in supervising medical and nursing staff in the psychological care of patients and in helping more directly in the management of psychiatrically complicated cases [*Stedeford and Bloch*,

1979]. The psychotherapeutic aspects of the care of these 49 patients were examined in detail. Their differing ways of coping with the stress of dying and the range of psychotherapeutic strategies used in treatment were described [*Stedeford*, 1979].

In addition to the research reviewed above, other studies have been concerned with the psychological consequences of mastectomy [*Maguire* et al., 1978], psychosexual problems in a venereal disease clinic [*Catalan* et al., 1981], and the nature and frequency of psychiatric morbidity in a physical rehabilitation hospital [*Holland and Whalley*, 1981].

### Research in Psychiatric Aspects of Obstetrics and Gynaecology

Several related studies have been carried out. These can be illustrated by two examples.

*Psychiatric Aspects of Hysterectomy.* 156 women with menorrhagia of benign origin were interviewed before hysterectomy, and re-interviewed 6 months post-operatively (n = 147) and again 18 months post-operatively (n = 148). Levels of psychiatric morbidity were significantly higher before the operation than after. On the Present State Examination, 58% of the patients were psychiatric cases before surgery, as against 29% at the 18-month follow-up. Similar post-operative improvements were found on measures of mood (Profile of Mood State) and of psychosexual and social functioning. Most of these improvements had occurred within 3–6 months after the operation. Both before and after hysterectomy, levels of psychiatric morbidity were high by comparison with women in the general population but lower than in psychiatric patients. The pre-operative psychiatric morbidity had been mainly of long duration. Psychiatric outcome was strongly associated with pre-operative mental state, neuroticism, previous psychiatric history, and family psychiatric history. No psychiatric differences were found between patients who had organic pathology in the uterus and those who did not, nor between patients who received bilateral oophorectomy and those who did not [*Gath* et al., 1982a, b].

*Psychiatric Sequelae to Interval Elective Sterilization in Women.* In a study of 201 women undergoing elective interval sterilization, there was no evidence that the operation led to psychiatric disorder. Pre-operatively the prevalence of psychiatric morbidity as measured by the Present State Examination was 10.4%, no greater than might be expected in a general population sample, 6 months after surgery the prevalence was significantly reduced to 4.7%, and 18 months post-operatively it had returned to 9.3%, slightly under the pre-operative level. Post-operative psychosexual disturbances was rare. Considerable regret was reported by only 2.6% 6 months after surgery, and by 4.1% 18 months after. Post-operative psychiatric disturbance and dissatisfaction were largely associated with pre-operative psychiatric disturbance [*Cooper* et al., 1982a].

Other psychiatric studies of gynaecological conditions include: the psychological and social determinants of pre-menstrual tension; the nature, frequency and aetiology of 'maternity blues' and of affective disorders occurring in the year following childbirth; a community survey of the nature, frequency and inter-relationships of psychiatric disorders and gynaecological disorders in women aged 30–65, with special reference to pre-menstrual tension, menorrhagia, and the menopause.

### Research on Deliberate Self-Harm

Since 1972 research has been carried out on epidemiological and clinical aspects of patients admitted to the general hospital for deliberate self-harm. In a series of epidemiological studies trends of self-poisoning and self-injury have been monitored [*Bancroft* et al., 1975; *Hawton* et al., 1982]. In the 10 years to April 1973 a fourfold increase in the incidence of deliberate self-harm occurred in Oxford City. Thereafter further increases occurred until the late 70s when there was a small decline. Amongst deliberate self-harm patients there are consistent patterns over the years. Females always outnumber males. Just over two thirds of all subjects are under 35 years of age, the rate being especially high for girls in their late teens and males in their late 20s. Almost 90% of admissions to the general hospital are for self-poisoning. Analysis of the substances used for self-poisoning over the years shows a marked decrease in the use of barbiturates, and an increase in the use of non-prescribed analgesics, especially paracetamol. Currently analgesics and minor tranquillisers are the substances most commonly used in overdoses. Other studies have examined the social and psychological characteristics of deliberate self-harm patients in general, and of particular subgroups, such as adolescents, students, epileptics, and people who repeat deliberate self-harm.

Another group of studies were concerned with attitudes towards deliberate self-harm. For example, in a study of general hospital staff [*Ramon* et al., 1975] it was found that physicians were far less sympathetic than nurses towards deliberate self-harm patients. However, physicians showed more sympathy to patients whose deliberate self-harm appeared to be associated with serious suicidal intent. It was also found that psychiatrists were more sympathetic than physicians [*Hawton* et al., 1981b].

Several studies have been concerned with the treatment of deliberate self-harm [*Hawton and Catalan*, 1982]. For example a comparison of nursing staff and psychiatrists, all of whom had undergone similar training in assessment procedures, showed that nurses were able to carry out assessments of deliberate self-harm as reliably as the doctors [*Catalan* et al., 1980]. Another study compared the effectiveness of domiciliary treatment and of out-patient care for deliberate self-harm patients [*Hawton* et al., 1981a]. Domiciliary care resulted in greater compliance with treatment, but was no more effective in improving mood, social adjustment, problem resolution or repetition of attempts.

## Conclusions

In this last section we have reviewed some examples of research into consultation-liaison in Oxford. We believe that these examples indicate the principal themes of research in the United Kingdom as a whole. The references on deliberate self-harm and the conference report of the Society for Psychosomatic Research [1981] provide further illustrations of the range of research interests.

## References

Association of University Teachers of Psychiatry: Working paper for conference on recruitment into psychiatry (1982).

Bancroft, J.; Skrimshire, A.; Reynolds, F.; Simkin, S.; Smith, J.: Self-poisoning and self-injury in the Oxford area: epidemiological aspects 1969–73. Br. J. prev. soc. Med. *29:* 170–177 (1975).

Brooks, P.; Walton, H.J.: Liaison psychiatry in Scotland. Health Bull. *39:* 218–227 (1981).

Catalan, J.; Bradley, M.; Gallwey, J.; Hawton, K.: Sexual dysfunction and psychiatric morbidity in patients attending a clinic for sexually transmitted diseases. Br. J. Psychiat. *138:* 292–296 (1981).

Catalan, J.; Marsack, P.; Hawton, K.E.; Whitwell, D.; Fagg, J.; Bancroft, J.H.H.: Comparison of doctors and nurses in the assessment of deliberate self-poisoning patients. Psychol. Med. *10:* 483–491 (1980).

Cooper, P.; Gath, D.; Rose, N.; Fieldsend, R.: Psychological sequelae to elective sterilisation: a prospective study. Br. med. J. *284:* 461–464 (1982a).

Cooper, P.; Osborn, M.; Gath, D.; Feggetter, G.: Evaluation of a modified self-report measure of social adjustment. Br. J. Psychiat. *141:* 68–75 (1982b).

Crisp, A.: The role of the psychiatrist in the general hospital. Post-grad. med. J. *44:* 267–276 (1968).

Editorial: Psychiatry in the general hospital. Br. med. J. *282:* 1256–1257 (1981).

Fleminger, J.J.; Mallett, B.L.: Psychiatric referrals from medical and surgical wards. J. ment. Sci. *108:* 183–190 (1962).

Gath, D.; Cooper, P.; Bond, A.; Edmonds, G.: Hysterectomy and psychiatric disorder. II. Demographic psychiatric and physical factors in relation to psychiatric outcome. Br. J. Psychiat. *140:* 342–350 (1982a).

Gath, D.; Cooper, P.; Day, A.: Hysterectomy and psychiatric disorder. I. Levels of psychiatric morbidity before and after hysterectomy. Br. J. Psychiat. *140:* 335–342 (1982b).

Goldberg, D.: The detection of psychiatric illness by questionnaire (Oxford University Press, London 1972).

Goldberg, D.P.; Cooper, B.; Eastwood, M.R.; Kedward, H.B.; Shepherd, M.A.: A standardised psychiatric interview for use in community surveys. Br. J. prev. soc. Med. *24:* 18 (1970).

Hawton, K.E.: Long-term outcome of psychiatric morbidity detected in general medical patients. J. psychosom. Res. *25:* 237–243 (1981).

Hawton, K.E.; Bancroft, J.; Catalan, J.; Kingston, B.; Stedeford, A.; Welch, N.: Domiciliary and out-patient treatment of self-poisoning patients by medical and non-medical staff. Psychol. Med. *11:* 169–177 (1981).

Hawton, K.E.; Catalan, J.P.: Attempted suicide: a practical guide to its nature and management (Oxford University Press, Oxford 1982).

Hawton, K.E.; Fagg, J.; Marsack, P.: The attitudes of psychiatrists to deliberate self-poisoning: comparison with physician and nurses. Br. J. med. Psychol. *54:* 341–347 (1981b).

Hawton, K.E.; Fagg, J.; Marsack, P.; Wells, P.: Deliberate self-poisoning and self-injury in the Oxford area 1972–80. Soc. Psychiatr. *17:* 175–179 (1982).

Hawton, K.E.; Gath, D.; Smith, E.: Management of attempted suicide in Oxford. Br. med. J. *ii:* 1040–1042 (1979).

Holland, L.K.; Whalley, M.J.: The work of the psychiatrist in a rehabilitation hospital. Br. J. Psychiat. *138:* 222–229 (1981).

Kenyon, F.E.; Rutter, M.: The psychiatrist and the general hospital. Compreh. Psychiat. *4:* 80–89 (1963).

Lloyd, G.: Whence and whither liaison psychiatry. Psychol. Med. *10:* 11–14 (1980).

MacLeod, J.; Walton, H.: Liaison between physicians and psychiatrists in a teaching hospital. Lancet *ii:* 789–792 (1969).

Maguire, G.P.; Julier, D.L.; Hawton, K.E.; Bancroft, J.H.J.: Psychiatric morbidity and referral on two general medical wards. Br. med. J. *i:* 268–270 (1974).

Maguire, G.P.; Lee, E.G.; Bevington, D.J.; Kuchemann, C.S.; Crabtree, R.J.; Cornell, C.E.: Psychiatric problems in the first year after mastectomy. Br. med. J. *i:* 963–965 (1978).

Mayou, R.A.: Psychological reactions to myocardial infarction. J. R. Coll. Physicians *13:* 103–105 (1979).

Mayou, R.A.; MacMahon, D.; Sleight, P.; Florencio, M.J.: Early rehabilitation after myocardial infarction. Lancet *ii:* 1399–1402 (1981).

Mezey, A.; Kellet, J.: Reasons against referral to the psychiatrist. Post-grad. med. J. *47:* 315–319 (1971).

Ramon, S.; Bancroft, J.M.J.; Skrimshire, A.M.: Attitudes towards self-poisoning among physicians and nurses in a general hospital. Br. J. Psychiat. *127:* 257–264 (1975).

Shepherd, M.; Davies, B.; Culpan, R.H.: Psychiatric illness in the general hospital. Acta psychiat. neurol. scand. *35:* 518–525 (1960).

Society for Psychosomatic Research: J. psychosom. Res. *25:* 323-476 (1981).

Stedeford, A.: Psychotherapy of the dying patient. Br. J. Psychiat. *135:* 7–14 (1979).

Stedeford, A.; Bloch, S.: The psychiatrist in the terminal care unit. Br. J. Psychiat. *135:* 1–6 (1979).

Stengel, E.: Suicide and attempted suicide (Penguin, London 1964).

Wing, J.K.; Cooper, J.E.; Sartorious, N.: The measurement and classification of psychiatric symptoms (Cambridge University Press, London 1974).

D. Gath, MD, University Department of Psychiatry,
Warneford Hospital, Oxford (England)

Adv. psychosom. Med., vol. 11, pp. 127–132 (Karger, Basel 1983)

# Consultation-Liaison Psychiatry in Japan

*Hitoshi Ishikawa*

Department of Psychosomatic Medicine, Tokyo University Branch Hospital, Tokyo, Japan

## Introduction

Consultation-liaison psychiatry is in a relatively young phase of development in Japan. My discussion comes from both a personal perspective as well as the historical development.

Orthodox Japanese psychiatrists are generally less concerned with problems at the interface between medicine and psychiatry than their counterparts in the United States. Their main interest lies in the diagnosis and treatment of psychiatric disorders such as schizophrenia and depression. Due to this focus, there has been little energy or interest in developing programs that interdigitate with clinical medical sciences such as internal medicine, pediatrics or gynecology. This situation is reflected by the small number of individuals who primarily practice consultation-liaison psychiatry. These individuals are usually found in university hospitals. Another indication of the minimal interest in this subspecialty is the paucity of professional organizations that relate to and promote consultation-liaison activities.

## History of Consultation-Liaison Psychiatry

The historical development of consultative psychiatry and liaison activities endeavors within Japan has been a slow and arduous task. Consultative psychiatry has developed far more than liaison activities. With a traditional psychiatric approach on diagnosis and treatment, the psychiatrist in Japan who performs consultative psychiatry will frequently be called to see acute psychotic disturbances within the internal medicine, pediatric or surgical wards. This is in contradistinction to the United States where consultation and liaison activities have made great strides with generous financial funding from the National Institutes of Mental Health. Liaison psychiatry has made even less of an impact in Japan than consultative work. The team approach, implicit in liaison work with medical units, has been underdeveloped in Japan. Furthermore, liaison psychiatry tends to espouse an integrated approach of psychosocial care which is prone to oversimplification and imprecisely called the psychosomatic approach. The psychosomaticist in Japan has been the general practitioner, internist, pediatrician or gynecologist rather than the psychiatrist. Thus, liaison psychiatry has not developed but, instead, a group of nonpsychiatric physicians who view themselves as 'psychosomaticists' has emerged.

### Operational Role of Consultation and Liaison Activities in Japan

Psychiatric consultations are widely available within Japan. The consultation, however, has a traditional function as the psychiatrist is asked to assess an identified psychiatric patient with an axis 1 disorder (DSM III) within a general medical setting. The descriptive approach utilized in these settings does not often emphasize detection of subclinical states or axis 2 disorders (DSM III).

Psychiatric consultation in ambulatory clinics is less well developed as psychiatrists have restricted their activities far more to hospital settings. Individuals who perform such consultative activities in outpatient settings are often 'psychosomaticists', and are physicians with training in internal medicine, pediatrics or gynecology. Japanese psychiatrists have traditionally had little interest in working with patients with traditional psychosomatic disorders such as peptic ulcer disease, asthma or situations where emotional and organic factors seem to interplay.

### Present Consultation-Liaison Activities in Japan

Despite the above difficulties which have resulted in this slow development, a small group of pioneer psychiatrists began to work within medical settings. Our present situation is parallel to consultation-liaison activities in the 1950 swithin the United States. It is interesting that those psychiatrists as well as other physicians who consider psychodynamic approaches to understanding behavior as important have become leaders in consultation-liaison work.i Psychoanalytic and psychodynamic approaches to behavior were introduced from the United States when a small group of Japanese psychiatric leaders returned from training within the United States. *Doi, Ninohara* and *Ikemi* laid the foundations for psychosomatic medicine in Japan. These individuals and their students, however, provided a unique integration of psychodynamic approaches with other theoretical systems. For example, *Ikemi* et al. [1] and *Ikemi and Ishikawa* [2] utilized three integrated approaches to their patient population. Autogenic training, transactional analysis and behavioral therapy were utilized in patients with various symptomatic states. The majority of patients receive autogenic training initially. Patients with neuromuscular disturbances or compulsive tics receive biofeedback training whereas patients with anxiety complaints or compulsive neurotic symptoms undergo behavioral treatment, primarily systematic desensitization. Those individuals who are felt to have underlying psychodynamic conflicts that create more character pathology than overt symptoms receive transactional analysis or Gestalt therapy. *Ishikawa* [3] extended this approach further and attempted to integrate these three treatment approaches utilizing cybernation therapy. Thus, the very early pioneers in consultation-liaison psychiatry within Japan utilized psychodynamic treatments in a monolithic fashion but soon were influenced by other theoretical approaches and attempted to integrate behavioral therapy and other learning theory paradigms into a more global approach.

*Nagakawa and Ikemi* [4] have recently reviewed the evolution of Japanese psychosomatic theory. As noted, interpersonal and individual psychodynamic psychologies are due to occidental influence from Japanese psychiatrists who trained in the United States. Other approaches such as autogenic training, biofeedback and meditation are distinctly syntonic with oriental culture. By integrating these theoretical paradigms, a comprehensive model has been developed utilizing a hierarchical development of stresses and appropriate therapies. Thus, treatment goals range from strategies to treat individual existential anxiety or characterologic problems and evolve into tactics to treat situational stress and somatic dysfunction which are best managed by biofeedback and direct counseling. Difficulties which constitute the existential and characterologic problems are best managed by insight-oriented and humanistic psychological approaches.

It must also be emphasized that utilization of dynamic techniques have been tailored to conform with the cultural and developmental parameters of Japan. Thus, transactional analysis which is frequently utilized within Japan has been modified by *Ikemi and Sugita* [5] to be more conducive to the Japanese cultural and developmental parameters. In view of the parent-adult-child classification utilized in the United States, these investigators modified this approach to view interpersonal transactions as 'heart-to-heart sincere transactions; social or technical transactions; defensive transactions and periphrastic transactions'. These classifications are far more appropriate than the American version of 'games' which in Japan connotes tactical crafty transactions.

## Research

The research activities of Japanese psychosomaticists include a broad range of endeavors. *Nakagawa* et al. [6] have looked at the epidemiology of depression within a population of internal medicine patients. They have also attempted to correlate gastric physiology with affective changes. Clinical investigations have included innovative approaches to the treatment of hysterical blindness utilizing behavioral therapy [7]. Utilizing an integrated approach of behavioral and psychodynamic approaches, *Ikemi* et al. [8] have been able to reduce stress in a group of chronic asthmatics. Thus, the Japanese psychosomaticists are continuing to demonstrate the importance of mind-body interactions in their research. The practical and clinical significance of this work will hopefully stimulate practitioners to give more attention to the tenets of our discipline.

## Future Trends

Consultation-liaison psychiatry has been slow to develop in Japan when compared to the United States. The lack of reimbursement for psychiatric care, the minimal interest in psychosomatic medicine by orthodox psychiatry, and the underrecognition of the efficacy of psychiatric consultation by family physicians causes this slow growth. The health insurance system in Japan generously rewards technologic procedures but neglects the psychological aspects of medical care. Specifically, there is poor reimbursement for psychiatric consultative services. Thus, both on the intellectual level as well as the material level little attention has been paid to the psychological aspects of medical care in the national health insurance reimbursement plans.

There are many obstacles be to overcome if consultation-liaison psychiatry is to flourish in Japan. The first step is to stimulate consultation-liaison activities among general psychiatrists and concurrently foster more psychological understanding among family practitioners. This will take major educational and organizational efforts by the present consultation-liaison groups in Japan. Development of psychosomatic societies may help this goal [9]. As medical practice is sharply demarcated between specialties, it will take a major effort to allow fluidity in consultation efforts to be developed between medical and psychological services. In addition to cognitive and intellectual factors, there needs to be a fundamental change in the entire medical system for consultation-liaison psychiatry to be a major element in medical care in Japan. Because relatively few consultations are performed in our medical system, the relationship between consultant and patient is difficult. General practitioners consulting with psychiatrists are often reluctant to take the initiative or responsibility for their recommendations. This leaves the consultant psychiatrist with difficult cases that have been 'passed on to the specialist'. Because of this, psychiatrists are faced with an excessive burden as a result of consultative activities. This helps explain their tendency to avoid doing consultative duties. By developing a more interdisciplinary approach, as found in consultation-liaison psychiatry, this problem may be overcome.

A basic strategy to overcoming problems both in organization in medical practice, attitudes which are nonpsychiatric, and developing more personnel, may be medical education. All medical colleges in Japan have psychiatric departments which include consultation-liaison psychiatry in their basic lectures. Six of the medical schools also have departments of psychosomatic medicine which offer more organized courses on the discipline. Postgraduate fellowships are available in psychosomatic medicine departments for training in psychosomatic areas. Within departments of psychiatry, training in consultation-liaison psychiatry is also available. In addition, the Japanese Society of Psychosomatic Medicine offers postgraduate lecture courses for general practitioners several times a year. With this amount of activity, the academic level achieved by the psychosomatic divisions is excellent. At the present time, however, most Japanese schools of medicine do not have independent departments designated for psychosomatic medicine. Only four national universities and two private colleges of medicine have defined departments for psychosomatic medicine. Even within these settings, budgets and staffs are insufficient. The paucity of resources reflects the common attitude of the Japanese medical world in general and family physicians in particular to underestimate the need for consultation-liaison psychiatry. One example of the neglect that the general medical field has for consultation-liaison activities is comprehensive care of terminal patients. Although this subject has been seriously undertaken in the United States and Europe, Japan has virtually nothing developed in comprehensive terminal care until very recently. Oriental religion has little bearing on medicine in Japan. We have largely abandoned traditional oriental medicine which was imbued with religion and instead adopted western technologic medicine which disassociates itself from religion. This has allowed medicine to focus only on the physical dimension, not on the psychological or social aspects of care. This peculiarity is due to the very rapid and excellent growth of technologic medicine. Unfortunately, psychosocial aspects have lagged behind. This may, in fact, be the most cogent explanation of the failure of Japan to properly integrate psychiatric care into medical care. It is the function of the consultation-liaison psychiatrist to abet this process.

## References

1  Ikemi, Y.; Ishikawa, H.; Goyeche, J.R.M.; Sasaki, Y.: Positive and negative aspects of the altered states of consciousness induced by autogenic training, zen and yoga. Psychother. Psychosom. *30:* 170–178 (1978).

2  Ikemi, Y.; Ishikawa, H.: Integration of occidental and oriental psychosomatic treatments. Psychother. Psychosom. *31:* 324–333 (1979).

3  Ishikawa, H.: Psychosomatic medicine and cybernetics. Psychother. Psychosom. *31:* 361–366 (1979).

4  Nakagawa, T.; Ikemi, Y.: A new model of integrating occidental and oriental approaches. J. psychosom. Res. *26:* 57–62 (1982).

5  Ikemi, Y.; Sugita, M.: The oriental version of transactional analysis. Psychosomatics *16:* 164–170 (1975).

6  Nakagawa, T.; Nagato, H.; Kimura, M.; et al.: A clinical and psychophysiological study of depression in internal medicine. Psychosomatics *17:* 173–179 (1976).

7  Ohno, Y.; Sugita, M.; Takeya, T.; et al.: The treatment of hysterical blindness by behavior therapy. Psychosomatics *15:* 79–82 (1974).

8  Ikemi, Y.; Nagata, S.; Ago, Y.; et al.: Self control over stress. J. psychosom. Res. *26:* 51–56 (1982).

9  McMahon, C.E.; Koppes, B.S.: The development of psychosomatic medicine: an analysis of growth of professional societies. Psychosomatics *17:* 185–188 (1976).

H. Ishikawa, MD, Department of Psychosomatic Medicine, Tokyo University Branch Hospital, 3-28-6, Mejirodai, Bunkyo-ku, Tokyo (Japan)

Adv. psychosom. Med., vol. 11, pp. 133–142 (Karger, Basel 1983)

# Consultation-Liaison Psychiatry in Italy

*Giovanni A. Fava, Luigi Pavan*[1]

Department of Psychiatry, State University of New York at Buffalo, N.Y., USA;
Chair of Psychiatry, University of Padua School of Medicine, Padua, Italy;
Institute of Psychology, University of Bologna School of Medicine, Bologna, Italy

Consultation-liaison psychiatry has a relatively recent history in Italy. The first papers on this topic started to appear in the 1970s in Italian medical journals and the first monograph was in 1976 [14]. There are essentially two reasons for this delay. First, only very recently has there been a separation of psychiatry from neurology in Italian academic settings and nonteaching hospitals; the obsolete model of the 'neuropsychiatrist' with its biological orientation has certainly delayed the development of psychosocial medicine. The psychiatric consultation was often called the 'neuro' consultation. Usually limited to severe psychiatric disorders, it was ideologically 'organic' in attitude. Second, psychosomatic medicine, which developed in Italy in the 1950s as a result of the efforts of *Ferruccio Antonelli* and other pioneers, initially developed outside of psychiatry and academic settings. Its orientation was strongly directed toward psychosocial aspects of general practice, after *Balint's* teaching. Therefore, the Italian psychiatry's interest in psychosomatic medicine is also recent.

Italy's revolutionary mental health law, which was passed in May 1978, but only recently started operating, has provided a dramatic impetus toward the development of consultation-liaison psychiatry. The gradual closing of the state psychiatric hospitals by first stopping all first admissions and then all readmissions, the institution of 15-bed units in each general hospital as the only form of psychiatric inpatient service and the formation of community-oriented mental health services, have led to an integration of psy-

[1] We are deeply indebted to *Marvin I. Herz*, MD and *George J. Molnar*, MD (State University of New York at Buffalo) and *Joan D. Koss*, PhD (University of New Mexico School of Medicine), for their helpful comments, and Ms. *Judy K. Deavers* for editorial assistance.

chiatry into medicine and to a transfer of state psychiatric hospitals staff to the general hospitals [12]. Medical wards have started managing patients who in the past would have been promptly transferred to psychiatric services and the role of consultation psychiatry has increased.

A recent meeting was dedicated to issues of consultation psychiatry in general hospitals in Italy; the first time such a meeting was held provides evidence for the emerging importance of this field [4].

Considering the different background and developmental patterns, a question of considerable interest is whether Italian consultation services differ from comparable American services. We will examine the clinical differences among three services relying on the data derived from three studies which were performed in the United States, Canada and Italy and employed similar methodologies. Cross-cultural differences will be emphasized through the description of the practical functioning of the Italian service which was studied and discussing the clinical implications of the data. Since the information concerning the Italian service was collected before the new mental health law (and no comparable information is available yet), we will also illustrate some possible future trends in consultation-liaison psychiatry in Italy.

### Cross-Cultural Differences in Consultation-Liaison Psychiatry

Until recently, discussions concerning the clinical activity of consultation-psychiatry services have been of a rather impressionistic and anecdotal nature. *Lipowski's* group reversed this trend by stressing the importance of the systematic collection of data on consultation activities. They studied 1,000 medical and surgical inpatients referred for psychiatric consultation at the Dartmouth-Hitchcock Medical Center in Hanover, N.H. [6]. *Taylor and Doody* [17] and *Fava and Pavan* [5] replicated the study in a Toronto hospital and in the University of Padua School of Medicine medical center. These studies, employing similar methodologies and diagnostic criteria, provide a solid basis for discussion of cross-cultural differences between consultation psychiatry in North American and Italian hospitals.

Table I shows that in all the consultation services the majority of referrals concern women and come from medical wards. There are very few differences in age between the American and Canadian samples. In the Italian patient population referred for consultation younger age is overrepresented: more than 60% of the patients are under 39 years of age against the approximately 40% of the North-American samples. One notes

Table I. Sex, age and source of referrals in consultation

| | Shevitz et al. [16] (n = 1,000) | Taylor and Doody [17] (n = 874) | Fava and Pavan [5] (n = 500) |
|---|---|---|---|
| Sex | | | |
| Male | 36.4 | 36.2 | 38.8 |
| Female | 63.6 | 63.8 | 61.2 |
| Age, years | | | |
| Under 19 | 5.0 | 4.8 | 13.2 |
| 20–29 | 17.3 | 21.6 | 28.0 |
| 30–39 | 17.0 | 13.6 | 22.8 |
| 40–49 | 17.4 | 13.7 | 11.6 |
| 50–59 | 17.8 | 16.1 | 11.0 |
| 60–69 | 15.8 | 15.6 | 10.2 |
| 70 and over | 9.7 | 14.6 | 3.2 |
| Source of referrals | | | |
| Medical | 79.0 | 65.0 | 75.8 |
| Surgical | 19.4 | 25.4 | 7.0 |
| Obstetric and gynecological | 1.1 | 9.6 | 8.2 |
| Others | 0.5 | – | 9.0 |

Results are expressed in percentages.

Table II. Primary psychiatric diagnoses in consultation

| DSM-II diagnosis | Shevitz et al. [16] (n = 1,000) | Taylor and Doody [17] (n = 874) | Fava and Pavan [5] (n = 500) |
|---|---|---|---|
| Depression | 50.2 | 36.8 | 37.0 |
| Organic brain syndrome | 15.5 | 18.8 | 1.6 |
| Anxiety neurosis | 6.8 | 5.8 | 18.6 |
| Hysterical neurosis, conversion type | 5.2 | 8.4 | 1.2 |
| Schizophrenia and paranoid psychoses | 3.1 | 4.5 | 3.2 |
| Alcoholism and drug dependence | 3.0 | 5.0 | 18.4 |
| Psychophysiological disorders | 1.9 | 3.7 | 6.0 |
| Others | 9.7 | 14.7 | 3.2 |
| No diagnosis | 4.6 | 2.3 | 10.8 |

Results are expressed in percentages.

also that surgery referrals represent 7% of the requests for consultation in the Padua Medical Center compared to the 19.4 and 25.9% of the North-American samples.

Table II reports the DSM-II diagnoses of the consultation services. Depression is the most common disorder in all samples and its prevalence in the Canadian and Italian samples is strikingly close. While, however, the American and Canadian populations referred for consultation show a similar trend for the other diagnostic categories, the Italian patient population shows distinctive diagnostic patterns.

Organic mental disorders are the second most common psychiatric disorder in the North American studies. However, there are only 1.6% such diagnoses in our sample. This may be due to the fact that in Italian hospitals patients with organic mental disorders are usually managed by medicine and surgery without any psychiatric support and referrals for their diagnosis and treatment are generally made to the Neurologic Consultation Service. The very low percentage of referrals for people aged 70 years or over (3.2%) in the Italian sample is consistent with this hypothesis, since it is in the elderly that organic mental disturbances predominate. It is held that Italian psychiatrists deal with the psychogenic – not with brain pathology. So it is not surprising that this area of psychiatry is largely neglected [5].

In the Italian sample the most common psychiatric diagnosis, after depression, is anxiety neurosis. It predominates in cardiovascular, dermatologic and musculoskeletal diseases. Alcoholism and/or drug dependence are the primary psychiatric diagnoses in 18.4% of cases. While alcoholism (4.6%) seems to be a major psychiatric problem in patients with concurrent medical diagnosis, drug dependence (13.8%) has a limited place there (3.8%), as the most frequent psychiatric diagnosis (55.4%) in the absence of medical diagnosis. This reflects the fact that no specific units for the management of substance-abuse disorders are available in the Italian general hospitals and that therefore these patients are generally referred to the medical wards.

No psychiatric diagnosis was made in 10.8% of cases in Italy, compared to 4.6% of cases in the US and 2.3% in Canada. This reflects a general attitude among Italian consultants to avoid labeling wherever possible. Hospital physicians, in fact, may attempt to scapegoat the patient by applying labels instead of dealing with problems of poor communication between staff and patients. The phenomenon is more frequently found in patients of low socioeconomic status with limited schooling. Italian psychiatrists tend to view these processes as sociocultural problems rather than health problems residing within individuals. By asserting a lack of mental disorder in the patient, the consultant tries to help correct against inadequate medical management, explaining to the physician who requested the consultation that the patient's difficulty is related to problems in the ward milieu.

This awareness of the negative social implications of labeling a patient with a psychiatric diagnosis has deep roots in Italian psychiatry, where a strong antinosological movement is present, attacking the conservative medical model to assert the primacy of social processes in the causation of mental disorders. The shortcomings of this antinosological approach, which may prevent a patient from receiving adequate medical attention, have eloquently been discussed by *Akiskal and McKinney* [1]. As a result, in Italy there is a tendency for psychiatrists to simply label referrals as inappropriate, offering no help in managing some patients. This results in poor patient care and implies a lack of responsibility on the part of the psychiatrist. However, this nosological reluctance also presents some positive implications. As part of each evaluation the consultant must decide whether or not a psychiatric illness is present and treatment indicated. In actual practice, however, American consultants tend to recommend treatment almost automatically as well as to make a diagnosis, without a careful consideration of its necessity or possible harmful effects [8].

The example of depression is appropriate. Here a decision concerning the pharmacotherapeutic treatment is often difficult, since unfortunately there is little research available to aid in this decision. The severity of symptoms or their primary/secondary nature are often considered to be grounds for clinical decisions [9]. Intensity of symptoms may be misleading, however. In a recent survey in a nonteaching hospital close to Padua, we found that about 25% of 325 inpatients admitted during a 1-week period presented on a self-rating scale depressive symptoms as severe as those of psychiatric patients with well-defined major depressive illness [7]. *Frances and Clarkin* [8], discussing the relative indications for no psychiatric treatment, stress the importance of identifying patients at risk for negative or no response and patients likely to have a spontaneous improvement. Although we have no follow-up data on those depressive inpatients, it is conceivable that these categories of patients may be present in a high percentage of cases in a general hospital, especially since most depressions in medical settings arise from the specific situation and psychological threats to which the medical inpatient is exposed [11]. A cautious attitude seems to be wise. The hospital setting may be the ideal setting for performing a dexamethasone suppression test, identifying those patients presenting a major depressive illness with features of melancholia [3]. This may avoid unnecessary pharmacotherapy potentially interacting with physical conditions or other forms of drug treatment.

### The Italian Consultation Psychiatric Service

The consultation service at the University of Padua School of Medicine operates in a 4,000-bed general teaching hospital which serves as one of the main referral centers for northeastern Italy. It is composed of 6 staff psychiatrists supervised by a senior psychiatrist (*L.P.*), who is also the psychiatrist-in-chief of the medical center. This situation is rather unusual in Italy and reflects his personal interest (generally there is a separate chief of the service). The 6 staff psychiatrists, as in most Italian teaching hospitals, are only on the service part-time, and also have ward or outpatient duties. Each psychiatrist covers a particular geographic area of the general hospital, which is therefore divided into six areas. The consultation requests go directly to the psychiatrist involved, according to the area of origin, and their acceptance does not follow a rotation schedule. This has the aim of encouraging the development of ongoing relationships between hospital physicians and consultants on the basis of mutual knowledge and work experience. Psychiatric residents and medical students do not rotate on the service but are encouraged to see some patients seen by its members. This is consistent with the general style of Italian medical consultation services (cardiology, gastroenterology, etc.), where only staff physicians assume consultation responsibility. Referrals are made by formal request from the hospital wards. There is no patient fee for the consultation, this being a covered benefit of the National Health Insurance System.

The population which is served by the consultation service has generally strong sociodemographic connotations, as we previously mentioned and as was shown by our survey on 500 consecutive referrals [5]. There is a preponderance of females, patients with a very low number of years of schooling (45.7% of the patients did not go over grade 5) and low social class (about 70% of the patients have a low socioeconomic status).

Housewives, people who are unemployed or have temporary jobs represent almost half of the sample. Social determinants seem to strongly influence the clinical diagnoses which were described in table II: people who live in urban settings tend to have a diagnosis of depression and drug dependence more often than rural residents, while those who live in rural areas are more frequently diagnosed as having anxiety neurosis and are more likely to be given no psychiatric diagnosis [5]. Seldom are upper class, highly educated patients referred for psychiatric consultation in our hospital, since psychiatric intervention in these cases is believed by physicians to be rejecting and offensive for the patient.

Lack of time is a major problem of the service. The fact that although the team is psychodynamically oriented treatment is solely pharmacotherapeutic in 58.2% of cases is highly indicative of this. A combination of psychotropic drugs and psychotherapy is used in about 16% of the cases, while other interventions (family therapy, psychotherapy only, etc.) are exceedingly rare. In 13.3% of cases no therapy is instituted.

Transfer of the patient to the psychiatric ward is seldom necessary, so that disposition problems are the source of the referrals in only 4% of the cases. Unfortunately, the department can provide neither beds for patients with combined medical and psychosocial problems nor ambulatory care services for the patients after they have been discharged from the hospital. The management of acutely psychotic patients on medical wards is generally recommended (this also reflects the spirit of the Italian mental health law). A relevant exception is found in patients with anorexia nervosa for whom a transfer to the psychiatric ward is almost preliminary to the consultation unless life-threatening and urgent medical problems are present. This reflects a long experience of the ward in dealing with anorectic patients and the conclusion that family therapy methods cannot be started when conflicts among physicians exist about the sick role designation (hospital physicians are generally reluctant to incorporate the family in the treatment program). Some preliminary data from a study we are undertaking on the follow-up of anorectic patients transferred to the psychiatric ward from the general hospital compared to those treated only on a medical ward by consultation psychiatry suggest the former group have a better outcome.

Psychosomatic research during consultation activities is strongly encouraged. A positive by-product is that it stimulates collaboration between consultants and hospital physicians. 5 out of the 6 staff psychiatrists in the service have at least one research project in the area of the hospital they cover. The survey on 500 referrals we previously mentioned provides further support for the view that research involvement on a unit stimulates the number and quality of referrals from the unit. At the time the study was done, an investigation concerning the psychological components of some dermatologic disorders [6] was in progress in the Institute of Dermatology, while no study was ongoing in the surgery units. It is interesting to observe how the dermatology unit, although composed of only a few dozen beds and referrals did not account for the research patients, had more requests for consultation than the surgical wards, which count several hundred beds [5].

### Future Trends in Consultation-Liaison Psychiatry in Italy

A discussion about the future of consultation-liaison psychiatry in Italy is inextricably linked to the outcome of the new Italian mental health law. Although its results seem to be positive [12] and a first report on the activity of a psychiatric consultation service in a general hospital is promising [2], it is too early for an assessment.

Certainly, the changes involved in the law have given strong impetus to consultative psychiatry. Nearly all psychiatrists working in general hospital or in community services are now called on to spend a part of their time in consultation activities; in the new National Health System mental health care is no longer geographically or conceptually separated from medical health care; the introduction of consultation activities outside the teaching hospital and at a community level could easily result in more comprehensive health care.

This quantitative growth of consultation psychiatry may not be translated, however, into a qualitative growth, in the sense of the introduction of psychosomatic concepts into practice. The model of consultative psychiatry prevalent in Italy today seems to be that defined by *Lipowski* [10] as the social reformist or community mental health model. It involves provision of assistance to health caregivers and promotion of mental health, a concept that this is laden with value judgements and lends itself to exploitation by political and special interest groups [10]. It contrasts with the psychiatric-therapeutic model, which entails provision of optimal care for the individual patient, his psychological status and his well being. The latter model was adopted in our psychiatric consultation service, where the consultant's role was well defined and restricted by his or her training, professional experience and skills. The fact that in Italy there is very little emphasis on teaching and training in consultation-liaison psychiatry may induce further confusion between the two models. Medical students and psychiatric residents may not be exposed at all to concepts of consultation-liaison psychiatry during their training; there are no postresidency fellowships in consultation psychiatry; the fact that psychiatric consultants in Italy are generally only part-time does not provide professional models likely to induce identification in younger professionals. Many psychiatrists who come from the state psychiatric hospitals and are now working in general hospitals may be unfamiliar with the concepts of psychiatry in a medical setting. There is considerable risk, therefore, that the psychosomatic needs of the medical services may remain unmet for lack of sufficient preparation both of the psychiatric consultants and of medical consumers.

It is not surprising that there is a growing interest among the Italian consultants who are interested in psychosomatic medicine toward liaison medicine as a way of practicing psychosomatic medicine [15]. We now have some evidence to support this view. We compared [*Pavan and Fava*, unpubl. data] 50 consultations provided by one of the authors within a liaison activity (involving weekly rounds) in a gastroenterology unit at the Padua Medical Center and 50 consultations provided at another time by the other author as part of the routine consultation activity on the same wards. Noteworthy differences in the two samples were present. First, the patients seen in consultation presented a very limited range of illnesses (ulcerative colitis, peptic ulcer, etc.), while those seen in liaison involved practically all type of gastrointestinal illness. Second, patients seen in liaison practice presented a significantly higher percentage of alexithymic traits than those referred for consultation, who, in turn, had a higher percentage of psychiatric diagnoses. Alexithymia is a relatively new concept to describe the impoverished fantasy life of some patients with somatic illnesses, with a resulting utilitarian way of thinking and a characteristic inability to use appropriate words to describe their emotions [13]. The importance of alexithymic phenomena in the production of somatic symptoms is well documented today [13]. It seems, therefore, that liaison medicine involves the incorporation of psychosocial issues in dealing with daily clinical problems such as alexithymia, instead of the pure management of the psychiatric complications of medical illnesses, or of the so-called 'psychosomatic diseases'. Consultation-liaison psychiatry in Italy, therefore, after a beginning inspired by American models of consultation psychiatry, seems to be also oriented now to the German model of psychosomatic medicine. The first chair of psychosomatic medicine was instituted at the University of Bologna School of Medicine a few years ago and it appears that others will follow, giving birth to services independent of psychiatry. At the same time, however, the social awareness of the Italian psychiatric consultants seems to be an innovative characteristic of the Italian model of consultation-liaison psychiatry and, in our opinion, deserves more attention than it received in the past, especially in North America, where, not surprisingly, data on the social characteristics of the samples seen in consultation seem to be lacking.

## References

1   Akiskal, H.S.; McKinney, W.Y.: Psychiatry and pseudopsychiatry. Archs gen. Psychiat. *28:* 367–373 (1973).

2   Bertolini, P.; Tansella, C.Z.; Tansella, M.: Attività di un servizio di psicologia medica in un ospedale generale. Riv. Psichiat. *14:* 413–422 (1979).

3   Carrol, B.J.; Feinberg, M.; Greden, J.F.; Tarika, J.; Albala, A.A.; Haskett, R.F.; McI. James, N.; Kronfol, Z.; Lohr, N.; Steiner, M.; de Vigne, J.P.; Young, E.: A specific laboratory test for the diagnosis of melancholia. Archs gen. Psychiat. *38:* 15–22 (1981).

4   Curci, P.; Rigatelli, M.: La consulenza psichiatrica nell'ospedale generale (Special issue). Riv. speri. Freniat. *105:* 256–423 (1981).

5   Fava, G.A.; Pavan, L.: Consultation psychiatry in an Italian general hospital. A report on 500 referrals. Gen. Hosp. Psychiat. *2:* 35–40 (1980).

6   Fava, G.A.; Perini, G.I.; Santonastaso, P.; Veller Fornasa, C.: Life events and psychological distress in dermatologic disorders. Br. J. med. Psychol. *53:* 277–282 (1980).

7   Fava, G.A.; Pilowsky, I.; Pierfederici, A.; Bernardi, M.; Pathak, D.: Depression and illness behavior in a general hospital. A prevalence study. VIth Int. Coll. Psychosom. Med., Montreal 1981.

8   Frances, A.; Clarkin, J.F.: No treatment as the prescription of choice. Archs gen. Psychiat. *38:* 542–545 (1981).

9   Gelenberg, A.J.: Antidepressants in the general hospital. Can. med. Ass. J. *120:* 1377–1385 (1979).

10  Lipowski, Z.J.: Psychiatric consultation. Concepts and controversies. Am. J. Psychiat. *134:* 523–528 (1977).

11  Moffic, H.S.; Paykel, E.S.: Depression in medical inpatients. Br. J. Psychiat. *126:* 346–353 (1975).

12  Mosher, L.R.: Italy's revolutionary mental health law. An assessment. Am. J. Psychiat. *139:* 199–203 (1982).

13  Nemiah, J.C.; Freyberger, H.; Sifneos, P.E.: Alexithymia; in Hill, Modern trends in psychosomatic medicine, part 3 (Butterworths, London 1976).

14  Pavan, L.: Lo psichiatra e lo psicologo nell'ospedale generale (Il Pensiero Scientifico, Roma 1976).

15  Rigatelli, M.; Curci, P.; DeBerardinis, M.: Some experiences of consultation-liaison psychiatry in a University hospital. Psychother. Psychosom. *33:* 1–6 (1980).

16  Shevitz, S.A.; Silberfarb, P.M.; Lipowski, Z.J.: Psychiatric consultations in a general hospital. A report on 1,000 referrals. Dis. nerv. Syst. *37:* 295–300 (1976).

17  Taylor, G.; Doody, K.: Psychiatric consultations in a Canadian general hospital. Can. J. Psychiat. *24:* 717–723 (1979).

G.A. Fava, MD, Research Assistant Professor, Department of Psychiatry,
State University of New York at Buffalo, Buffalo, NY 14215 (USA)

Adv. psychosom. Med., vol. 11, pp. 143–149 (Karger, Basel 1983)

# Consultation-Liaison Activities in Norway

*Finn Askevold*

Psychosomatic Division, The National Hospital, University of Oslo, Norway

## Introduction

Liaison psychiatry advances a psychobiosocial model into medicine. This is done by integrating the biographic anamnesis of each patient into their medical history. This allows understanding of how and to whom a disease affects. Delineation of the patient's personality and how he copes with the sick role in the context of his prior personal experience allows full integration of physical, psychological and social themes. The major challenge of psychosomatic medicine is how to best achieve this synthesis.

The success of consultation-liaison psychiatry in any country depends upon a number of separate factors. The economic realities of health care, the history and organization of psychiatry and the educational system all dictate the form of psychiatric care in general and the manner in which psychiatry is integrated into general medicine. The cultural acceptance of psychological factors in disease also becomes a crucial factor in allowing the emergence of consultation-liaison psychiatry. These factors may determine the strength of political advocacy for funding such interventions but cannot be substituted for the skill of liaison psychiatrists in demonstrating professional competence and communicating his needs to the individuals that determine funding patterns for health care.

## Consultation-Liaison Service in Norway: Special Aspects

The Norwegian society may, as other Scandinavian countries, be viewed as egalitarian. The backbone of its health service is the national insurance coverage which was established in 1967. It grants benefits in cases of illness, physical defects, pregnancy, childbirth, unemployment, old age, disablement, death and loss of income. It covers all persons living in Norway. The benefits for medical illness cover hospitalization, ancillary care and extended care facilities such as nursing homes.

Approved health institutions include hospitals, nursing homes, rehabilitation centers and recreation units. Funding is governed by the Ministry of Health and Welfare, Directory of Health, but the responsibility for erection, management and maintenance resides at a local county level, with a few exceptions where the government is the owner of the institution.

Several counties may merge into a region, thus, we have twenty counties and four regions. Each region has its teaching hospital. The Oslo region has two, one municipal and one federal, the single federal medical hospital in the country. Besides being highly specialized teaching hospitals, the regional hospitals also serve as the central hospital of the county of its location.

In the 20 counties of Norway there are 17 central hospitals, two counties are without such a facility and depend on the neighboring region hospital. Two counties, for geographical reasons, have more than one central hospital because the populations served are too extensive. In addition, there are 54 local hospitals in different communities. Their basic structures include three medical departments – surgery, medicine and radiology. Some local hospitals are more specialized, up to ten departments. The central hospitals have 10–20 specialties and service departments included, whereas the region hospitals have 20 to 35 departments.

In addition to, but separate from the general hospital, Norway has seven rehabilitation centers, four centers for orthopedic surgery, three for rheumatic disorders, three for pulmonary tuberculosis, one national cancer center and one geriatric hospital.

Psychiatric health institutions are excluded from the list above, as are institutions for treatment of alcohol and drug addicts. The psychiatric hospitals treat major mental disorders and are separate from the 'medical' hospital. Three of the general medical hospitals have included psychiatric treatment sections for minor psychiatric disorders within the facility. Ten central and three regional hospitals have a psychiatry department included in the general hospitals for minor psychiatric disorders. All departments have inpatient and ambulatory services. In three regional and five central hospitals, there are inpatient departments for child psychiatry and also outpatient departments. In an additional ten, there are outpatient services only, in child psychiatry.

*General Aspects – Liaison Endeavors*

*Norwegian Psychiatry*

Postwar psychiatry in Norway has been greatly influenced by psycho-dynamic theories and strategies. Hospital work has utilized therapeutic social environments and, when possible, has attempted to develop therapeutic communities, such as described by *Jones* [1]. Only in the last 5 years has behavioral therapy been actively included as a common therapeutic tactic. Psychiatry has been defined as a behavioral discipline in the past which fostered separation from general medicine. Present liaison efforts are attempting to reevaluate that position and develop a reapproachment to the medical sciences.

Psychiatric training within Norway begins following formal graduation from medical school. Nascient psychiatrists have a 5-year training program while working within psychiatric settings. Didactic training includes mandatory courses in addition to clinical experience and clinical supervision. Thus, psychiatric training within Norway is generally in institutions dedicated solely to the treatment of psychiatric problems. Liaison experience is gained within this 5-year program generally without formalized supervision. Only in our department at the Rikshospitalet is there a registrar's position that is dedicated to liaison work. In addition to the focused liaison experience, there is formalized supervision in this subspecialty.

Medical school education of psychiatry is primarily formal psychiatric diagnosis and evaluation. Eight lectures, however, are given in psychosomatic medicine in order to expose medical students to concepts of situations where medicine and psychiatry interface.

Development of a working alliance between psychiatry and medical disciplines depends on several factors.

*Geography*. Where the psychiatric service is situated several miles away from the somatic hospital it is self-evident that the old consultation model must be at work. The somatic department calls for consultations. In the psychiatric hospital this is received and handed out to one of the youngest and least experienced, who is sent to take a psychiatric interview, write his recommendation and disappear back to his ordinary work. He does nothing more unless the patient is admitted into the psychiatric hospital. One of our teaching hospitals has this situation, but because of disappointment, the department of social medicine has taken on the task of liaison work by its associate professor who is a specialist in psychiatry.

*Interest*. Even if there is a psychiatric department on the premises of the somatic hospital there is no guarantee that it will function beyond the level of consultation service. This depends on the degree of interest in the parts involved, but mostly on the psychiatrist. Medical education is still dominated by natural science and if the psychiatrists do not show themselves useful in other somatic cares than the pure psychiatric emergencies, they will be forgotten. They have to appear personally on the medical wards, learning to talk a language understandable to the staff and provide follow-up care to these patients. It is obvious that the psychiatrist in question must be one of the senior staff. Then it comes to the allotment of psychiatric resources.

In most of the hospitals there is no real liaison service. The reason is both lack of resources and lack of interest. The work load in the psychiatric department is as high as in the other departments. Psychiatry is a primary discipline in itself, so it is more just to say it is a question of priority of interest. Therefore, we must often utilize the consultation model at work. On the other hand, the level of interest, even if latent, varies in the medical hospitals least in the organ-centered, action-oriented departments such as surgery.

Usually, interest in psychological issues is greater in departments of medicine and neurology. There will, however, be collisions. As the cost-per-day increases, great emphasis is focused upon shortening the length of stay. This means careful coordination of diagnostic evaluation and therapeutic programs. In this context, it becomes difficult to squeeze in psychiatric interviews and even more problematic to offer a series of brief psycho-therapy sessions.

### Needs vs. Economy

The development of liaison services thus becomes basically a political question because it concerns distribution of the taxpayers' money to estab-lish liaison services. The group which has the least to say is the patients. It has been estimated a need for psychiatric advice concerning 30% of the patients on wards for internal medicine. This estimate is usually made by the doctors, but once the patient is aware of the possibility of a psychiatric consultation while on the medical ward an increasing number asks for one. Patients, however, are an unorganized group and do not have the capacity and power to put pressure on the politicians. Health personnel are better organized, but when it comes to making priorities on the budget, other medical departments do not feel that psychiatry is their responsibility and will not put liaison work on their priority list! Politicians depend on information from the health authorities for their allocation of money, thus liaison psychiatrists will end up far down in priority! If this discipline is to grow, the first step must be taken by the psychiatrists. They must share their resources with the medical departments and assign a permanent senior staff member for this task. Until the liaison psychiatrists have made themselves indispensable to medicine, the psychiatric department will need to expend its resources to offer liaison services. Then the liaison psychiatry will be seen as necessary and become the responsibility of the hospital administration, not of each department.

### The Actual Situation in Norway

Of the 54 local hospitals, two have psychiatrists on their staff without connection with the psychiatric departments. This happened both places because psychiatrists were available for private reasons. In six others, liaison work is carried out from the Department of Psychiatry and of Child Psychiatry. In the remaining 46 hospitals there is no such service.

In 10 out of 18 central hospitals there are departments of psychiatry and 8 for child psychiatry. In addition, there are 5 separate outpatient departments of child psychiatry in these hospitals. In 4 of the 5 regional teaching hospitals there are special liaison services. Mostly they are run by 1 person. Only in the National Hospital are there full-time liaison services both in the adult and the child area. In this institution the staffing includes two consultants and one registrar and a clinical psychologist on the adult service. The child service has one consultant and one registrar, a psychologist, a social worker and a teacher.

### Experience of Liaison Work

Only where the psychiatrist is located within a medical department can it be stated that a true liaison service exists. Thus, the experience of the National Hospital in Oslo, a 1,100 bed hospital with 30 departments, can be described.

The liaison service at the National Hospital has been in existence in its present form since 1959. During the 20 years, from 1960 to 1979, 7,253 patients, an almost equal number of males and females, have been seen. 50% are seen on the medical wards, 40% on the neurological wards and the remaining 10% on all the other wards. These figures represent 14% of all patients admitted to the medical wards and 10% of those on the neurological ward.

To estimate actual liaison needs of the hospital, we reviewed the records of all new patients during a 2-week period. The internists stated they wanted psychiatric help in 22% if there were no limit to psychiatric resources. We added another 10% from records only, and during the rounds we picked up an additional 4%, which makes a total of 36% in this medical department.

The diagnostic distribution was 43% pure psychiatric conditions, 22% psychosomatic disorders, 23% brain organic syndromes, 9% no demonstrable psychopathology and 3% were unclassifiable. Of the psychiatric disorders, neurotic reactions amounted to 60%, psychotic to 18%, depressions of nonpsychotic nature to 16% and neurasthenic reactions to 6%. Of the neurotics, 60% were conversion reactions, many of the old, classical type which, by many psychiatrists, is said to have disappeared in our present 'sophisticated' society. 30% were anxiety reactions and 10% obsessional states.

This clinical sample shows the varied picture from clear-cut psychiatric disorders with no organic disturbances to the psychosomatic syndromes with serious somatic conditions that coalesce with an intricate psychosocial interaction.

Of the referrals, 76% were for comprehensive diagnostic evaluation to help in treatment planning; 13% were for pure psychiatric symptoms, two-thirds of this being psychotic behavior, and 11% were legal or insurance cases, mostly disablement pensions in war veterans and concentration camp survivors. As the hospital is a tertiary care facility, it receives most of the patients from other hospitals. There are practically no emergencies, such as suicide attempts, intoxications or traffic accidents and no admissions for senile deterioration in need only of nursing. Thus, the composition of patients will differ from most other hospitals and consequently the liaison work will also be different. In comparison, the case load of a liaison service in a nearby municipal hospital revealed that 30% of their cases were for attempted suicide and another 30% were related to geriatric problems. In contradistinction, the National Hospital's liaison service saw no suicidal gestures and only had 1% of their cases devoted to geriatric problems. Thus, the tasks involved for the National Hospital's liaison service were more commonly collaborative efforts with medical colleagues rather than pure psychiatric management or dispositional problems. Only the direct contact with paitents is described above and represents merely one aspect of the liaison work.

Weekly conferences with the colleagues from the other departments are held to discuss the treatment aspects, both of patients seen directly and of those which they want our advice on, but where they take the full responsibility themselves.

With the other departments we communicate directly with the referring doctors. Both ways are creating an understanding of liaison work, and of social and psychological aspects of human disease and thus have an important teaching function.

With the nursing staff our relationship is less formal. It takes place on the wards or on the ward rounds.

Collaboration in research often takes place on selected topics. To give one example: the demonstration that the so-called whiplash damages give origin to organic brain damage; another is the work on the health sequences of the concentration camp survivors where neurology, neuroradiology, internal medicine, social medicine, neuropsychology and psychiatry collaborated to demonstrate the presence of a distinct concentration camp syndrome, now recognized all over the world.

## Conclusions

In many places in Norway the liaison work has not developed beyond the level of mere consultation practice. In isolated hospitals we have full-time liaison workers, but often it is a single-handed job without the backing of a liaison milieu. Only in a few places is there a developed liaison service, even if the capacity does not reach the level of need. There is still a long range to cover from 14% actually seen to the estimated 36% of needs.

To increase liaison services, resources initially have to be delegated from the psychiatric field. Only where the liaison workers have made themselves indispensable will their funding then be the responsibility of the administrators of the somatic hospitals. This will happen first in teaching hospitals and will evolve from them to central hospitals and some of the larger, local hospitals, and only then may we say that there are developed liaison services in Norway.

## Reference

1    Jones, M.: Social psychiatry (Tavistock Publications Ltd., London 1952).

F. Askevold, MD, Psychosomatic Division, The National Hospital,
University of Oslo, Oslo (Norway)

Adv. psychosom. Med., vol. 11, pp. 150–163 (Karger, Basel 1983)

# Consultation-Liaison Psychiatry in Belgium

*R.A. Pierloot, P. Nijs*

Department of Psychiatry, University of Leuven, Belgium

The 'psychosomatic movement' in Belgium, during the past 30 years, is characterized by a slow but progressive expansion from a few University hospitals to a large number of general hospitals and into general practice. Originally it was limited to the clinical service and research in consultation-liaison psychiatry at the University centers of Leuven, Brussels and Liège. Recently, the majority of general hospitals have developed some form of consultative psychiatry. Fully elaborated liaison medicine, however, remains rather exceptional. At the same time, a growing interest in psychosocial problems in medical practice has stimulated a number of general practitioners to seek postgraduate training in psychosocial topics or collaboration with psychiatrists and/or psychologists. This has resulted in the development of Balint groups; acquisition of skills in techniques of psychotherapy (relaxation, supportive therapy, counseling, etc.) by general practitioners and, in exceptional cases, the integration of a psychologist and/or social worker in a group general practice.

## General Overview: Consultation-Liaison in Belgium

At the University of Leuven, consultation-liaison psychiatry started within the Department of Internal Medicine of St. Rafaël hospital. In that department, *R. Pierloot*, having finished a training in internal medicine and completing his training in psychiatry, was appointed as a 'consultant on psychosomatics' in 1953. Having a physician trained in both psychiatry and medicine was unique. This allowed a psychosocial resource within a general hospital. Before 1953 most general hospitals had neither a psychiatric unit nor psychiatrists for consultation. Even today most hospitals in Belgium limit their psychiatric activities to an outpatient clinic. The majority of consultation-liaison work remains primarily in the academic centers described below.

During several years a number of patients, selected on the basis of their symptomatology (the so-called psychosomatic diseases, e.g. asthma, peptic ulcer) or/and manifest psychosocial problems were demonstrated to benefit by a multidisciplinary approach. This included psychological, social and somatic factors in an integrated manner [38–40, 44]. Residents and undergraduate medical students, during their training in internal medicine, became familiar with this approach. A number of research studies in the area of psychosomatics resulted from this clinical work [8–11, 41–43, 45–49, 51–53]. As the expansion of the Internal Medicine Department expanded due to subspecialization, specialized units (respiratory diseases, cardiology, gastroenterology, etc.) were established and hampered this type of collaboration. This subspecialization entailed a predominance of technical and laboratory procedures that outstripped the interest in psychosocial factors. In 1963, the psychiatric liaison facilities were transformed into an autonomous psychiatric outpatient department, functioning as a consultation service for the total hospital. This allowed a growing propagation of consultative psychiatry in the hospital. At the same time this new department offered opportunities for psychiatric residents to gain experience with psychiatric problems in different departments of a general hospital. Although the more formal liaison connections with the department of internal medicine no longer existed, collaboration on a consultative basis was maintained. In this milieu, new initiatives of liaison psychiatry arose. At the University rehabilitation hospital Pellenberg, that tests respiratory diseases, cardiology, rheumatology, and orthopedics, a liaison team consisting of a psychiatric resident, a trained psychiatrist and a psychologist have been developed. This liaison-consultative service now has 4 members: the staff psychiatrist *(B. Van Houdenhove)*, a part-time assistant psychiatrist, a staff psychologist and a student in clinical psychology. Their activities embrace diagnostic psychiatric evaluation as well as psychotherapy for selected patients and 'psychological coaching of the nursing staff' [55].

In the Department of Gynecology of St. Rafaël hospital, the liaison psychiatry activities started with the appointment of a full-time psychiatrist *(P. Nijs)* in 1968. The activities within this department can be regarded as the best example of an elaborated liaison psychiatry system; they will be described in detail below.

At the University of Brussels, regular consultative psychiatry activities have been developed at the Brugman hospital from 1955 by *D. Luminet* and *S. Cosyns-Duret*. Their activities have been elaborated mainly in connection with the departments of internal medicine and gynecology; a large number of psychosomatic research studies resulted from this work [2, 4–7, 12–19]. In 1974, *Luminet* moved to the University of Liège but consultative psychiatry continues under the direction of *Cosyns-Duret*.

At the University of Liège, the development of consultative psychiatry has been encouraged by the appointment of *M. Dongier* as professor of psychiatry in 1963. Psychiatrists in training became responsible for regular consultative duties in the different departments of the Bavière hospital. After the departure of *Dongier* in 1974, these consultative-liaison psychiatry activities have been promoted further by his successor, *Luminet* [20–22]. The department of internal medicine and dermatology of the Bavière hospital now possess their own psychiatrist.

At the University of Ghent, consultation-liaison started only the last years at the new university hospital. Regular staff members of the department of psychiatry *(P. Jannes, M. van Moffart)* direct these activities.

Health insurance in Belgium is universal and reimburses patients, totally or in part, according to the type of procedure. The total health care delivery system is catalogued into a list of individual acts, with technical procedures preferred and taxed at different rates of reimbursement. Thus use of technical procedures is much more remunerative than the time and/or intellectual effort required from the physician. Activities, typical and necessary for a group oriented approach, such as joint meetings and case discussions are not considered for reimbursement. This seriously handicaps liaison psychiatry work, which can be considered for financial intervention only insofar as it can be translated in individual performances, still belonging to the lower rated medical acts.

*A Specific Liaison Service: Liaison Psychiatry at a Gynecology Department (University of Leuven, Hospital St. Rafaël)*

The 'birth' of a psychiatrist, permanently attached to the gynecology department (1968) emerged during the proliferation of oral contraceptives since 1962 [23–25, 27, 30, 33]. The reason for this 'birth' was that the gynecologist giving contraceptive advice encountered a growing number of psychosocial and sexual problems among his patients. In the beginning, the cooperation between gynecologist and psychiatrist was not easy. The psychiatrist, with his focus upon psychological suffering, arrived in a totally different world, i.e. the 'Promised Land' where lives the myth of the child. Moreover, he came from psychiatry, the contemplative branch of medicine, and arrived in a surgical setting, where therapy means activity. For some gynecologists the psychiatrist was a 'special' man: he did not do anything with his 'clean hands'. Afflicted with a 'constitutional weakness in his legs', the psychiatrist tried in vain to find a chair in this gynecological environment where all the work is done *upright*. Both, psychiatrist and gynecologist looked for a common ground in which to interact. The focus of each way changed, i.e. the medical-somatic model versus a dynamic-relational model to a human-biological one which encompassed biological, psychological and social themes.

The department is located in the gynecological ward of the hospital. The psychiatric staff forms a division of the larger gynecological-obstetrical department. Besides the psychiatrist, 'chef-de-clinique', the team consists of an educator sexologist and a social worker. Two experienced residents in neuropsychiatry form part of the team for 1 year. One resident in psychiatry and two psychologist-sexologists are engaged in a research program on high-risk pregnancies, artificial insemination donor sperm, and reversible sterilization. One student psychologist-sexologist is also trained during 1 year as a family therapist. The secretary of this division is part of the team of secretaries of the Gynecological and Obstetrical Department.

Although the orientation of the team is based on psychoanalytic theories, the treatment offered may be crisis intervention where therapy is short but intensive (one or two sessions a week for 3–9 months), especially in the case of marital and intergenerational problems. Sexual dysfunctions are treated with a behavioral approach containing several suggestive elements. In a collaborative effort with Prof. *Molinski* and his co-workers (Dusseldorf, FRG) a modification of the Masters and Johnson sex therapy was developed [35, 36].

Through the years there has been a shift in problems which this team treated. From oral contraceptives, sterilization, and abortion consultation requests shifted towards infertility problems (adoption and artificial insemination) [3, 28, 29, 31, 34] and reversible sterilization [32]. Family planning received a new meaning, not only the regulation of the number of children but also the quality of human reproduction became important (e.g. artificial insemination when one partner of a couple is the carrier of a chromosomal deviation). This shift fostered development of an interdisciplinary team of counseling, consisting of gynecologists, an endocrinologist, an urologist, a psychiatrist and a medical ethicist. They formed a new unit: Human Fertility and Sterility [1].

Our approach to infertility problems has been influenced by *Balint's* 'The Doctor, The Patient and His Illness'. Members from our interdisciplinary team work with the infertile couple to reorganize their complaint. Human infertility is not viewed as a disease but a problem which is evaluated and hopefully solved by the couple as well as the medical team. An effort is made not to single out one member of the couple as the dysfunctional individual but to view the marital unit as the 'patient'. An attempt is made to allow open-ended dialogue to develop a full understanding of any specific difficulty in infertility. Thus, the consultation is characterized by joint clinical work and continuing didactic input so that the infertile couple may gain new knowledge about medical-technical, social-psychological and ethical issues. In order to make our interdisciplinary team an effective treatment vehicle, we have needed to allow a full 'willingness to listen'. Every member of this team has to free himself. This provides a basis for an interdisciplinary dialogue and a permanent 'training school' for a willingness to listen. Every member of this team has to free himself of potential biases due to his professional training, i.e. a narrow medical model, individualistic and organic, had to be changed to a relational approach of a couple with fertility or sexual problems. Moreover, the psychiatrist had to develop greater freedom from the psychoanalytical model which held the risk of hiding the psychosocial reality of the couple behind tempting fantasies. The point we looked for is a human-biological approach of human fertility and sexuality. There is a tension between the biological optimum of fertility and the human optimum of parenting. Man and wife are not mere coital instruments that should function adequately in a mechanical manner. Nor are they the mathematical sum of their chances of procreation. In this manner the course of Obstetrics at the Faculty of Medicine becomes a course in *human fertility* that is multidisciplinary using a gynecologist, obstetrician, endocrinologist, urologist and psychiatrist.

As noted this team is located in the gynecological and obstetrical clinic and the emphasis is on ambulatory care. Some 6,000 consultations a year are provided, financed following the rules of the Belgian National Health Insurance (psychiatric consultations). A positive balance makes the system financially viable. The very first patients were women referred by the gynecological clinic, originally for family planning (contraception or subfertility), later on for sexual and relational problems. Women with gynecological-psychosomatic problems – like chronic pelvic pain – constituted an equal number of patients. Gynecologists, specialists for internal diseases and general practitioners outside the hospital refer as well for the same problems. Patients also consult directly, especially for family planning and relationship problems. Working class people are somewhat underrepresented; most of the patients are middle class and to a less extent higher class. About 65% of the consultations are individual and 35% are conjoint consultations.

During our 10 years of experience, a satisfying integration has been developed. Therefore, this department was presented as a model on the 'Fortbildungstage für gynäkologische Psychosomatik' in Mainz (1978). Research topics of the department are: psychopathological aspects of oral contraception; reversibility of sterilization; sexuality and relationship during pregnancy. These research projects are financed by the Ministry of Health and the Family. Research on psychosocial and psychosomatic aspects of high risk pregnancies is also financed by the same ministry. Other important research projects are: psychopathological aspects of artificial insemination and chronic pelvic pain in women [37, 54]. A project on psychosomatic aspects of infertility or 'functional' infertility started only recently.

This model of integration in the gynecological clinic is also appreciated by gynecologists in the community, so that they are increasingly utilizing a psychologist for psychosocial problems. In the past decade, gynecological psychosomatics was extended to the gynecological clinic. For the future, the planning is to extend psychosomatic obstetrics. Therefore, a 2-year training course (a monthly meeting) was started for nursing staff. Based on the described multidisciplinary approach, a menopause clinic also started.

As stated before, the emphasis is on the ambulatory care. Yet hospitalization is sometimes needed: five beds on the gynecological ward are available for gynecological psychosomatic cases like anorexia nervosa or obstetrical problems like hyperemesis gravidarum and high risk pregnancies. [Editor's note: This is very different from Italy, cf. *Pavan and Fava's* chapter.]

*Consultation-Liaison Psychiatry in*
*Medical Education and Postgraduate Training*

A goal of establishing consultation-liaison activities is closely linked to the introduction of psychological, psychopathological and sociological concepts in medical education. The construction of physicochemical models has played a major role in medicine as a whole and has yielded important results.

The very success of this model, however, has increased the dangerous tendency for physicians to view illness as a physicochemical process alone. It is all the more imperative therefore that medical education provides the student with a counterpoint to allow him to understand the human experience of 'being ill' and its effects on the individual human being. In Belgium, as in many countries, it has become apparent that such a counterpoint must come from the introduction of psychological, sociological and psychiatric insights in medical education [50].

One of the primary tasks in medical education is to emphasize the fact that illness is more than a somatic process. No matter how important the physical aspects of an illness may be, being sick is a highly personal event for every patient, and the student must be made to see that the sick individual experiences his illness as something to be 'lived through' in the context of his human relationships. The physician is not merely a skilled technician, but is intimately involved in the patient's social network. Thus the physician must have both a theoretical knowledge of the nature of human relationships in general and a sensitivity to the nuances of the doctor-patient relationship itself.

The Belgian medical curriculum is 4 years in duration and may be entered only after a college program of 3 years that is especially aimed at the future study of medicine. Since the college program provides specific preparation for subsequent medical education, the curriculum includes lectures on psychology and sociology, which constitutes an introductory basis for the later study of medical psychology, psychopathology and psychiatry. This preparatory instruction is given in courses taught to large groups of students as passive listeners. In some of the colleges, this is complemented by small-group sessions in which students can discuss psychosocial topics related to illness and health care. Case histories can be reviewed or specific aspects of health services (e.g. crisis intervention, institutions for elderly people, self-help groups, etc.) are discussed. Students will also visit health care facilities. The choice of the topics is determined by the participants and in general, attendance to these small-group sessions is voluntary.

In teaching psychology and psychopathology we have shifted from the traditional concern with the phenomena of mental disorganization in psychotic conditions to greater interest in psychological and psychopathological adaptation reactions. Far more attention is paid to the detection of regressive and transference reactions, neurotic processes and disturbances related to psychosocial interactions than in the accurate delineation of the form of a delusion or the characteristics of a dementia. This necessitates different forms of teaching that make the student sensitive to the importance of emotional disturbance that could appear mild and benign on the surface but that may have profound repercussions in the patient's human functioning, and eventually lead to serious and lasting handicaps.

In essence the necessary basis for skills in consultation-liaison activities is knowledge about the more common and widespread reactions of the individual as he adapts to his psychosocial milieu. This changes the traditional teaching of psychopathology to seminars on personality development, ego defenses and the nature of transference in the doctor-patient relationship.

In the medical curriculum itself, teaching of psychiatry and its liaison aspects is offered under four forms: lectures, clinical demonstrations, small-group sessions and clinical clerkships. The lectures, usually given to large groups of students, contain basic areas of medical psychology and psychopathology. Lectures on clinical psychiatry are mostly illustrated by demonstration and discussion of case histories (by preference with video-taped material). In general, these are limited to rather typical psychiatric cases. Opportunities to introduce liaison psychiatry by discussing the same patient from different angles to study the medical, social and psychiatric points of view is done in only a few universities.

About 1½ years of the curriculum are reserved for clinical clerkships. Clerkships in internal medicine, surgery, pediatrics and obstetrics are obligatory, but psychiatry is optional. Besides the direct clinical contact with the patients, students attend small-group work meetings devoted to case discussions or/and expositions of clinical topics during these rotations. In contrast to the lectures, and clinical demonstrations, which are given almost exclusively by members of the permanent academic faculty, junior staff members are enlisted as instructors for the small-group exercises. This enables the student to gain a more diversified perspective on problems under consideration. At the same time he is led to a more active participation in his work through the greater ease with which he is able to relate to younger instructors. In this structure the opportunity to introduce liaison psychiatry depends on the attitude of the clinical department. In essence, liaison teaching requires a gracious 'host'.

Postgraduate training in psychiatry in Belgium is still combined with a training in neurology (3 years of residence in psychiatry, 2 years in neurology). Although it is not obligatory, the majority of the psychiatric residents spend 1 year in an outpatient department of a general hospital and offer consultative psychiatric service to other clinical departments. In the consultation-liaison service of gynecology, described above, experienced residents in neuropsychiatry are employed during 1 year, residents in gynecology have the possibility of a 6-month experience as part of their training program (gynecological psychosomatics and sexology). All members of the liaison department take part in the weekly staff conference on gynecology. A limited number, according to their own interests, takes part in the weekly staff seminar on fertility-sterility and high risk pregnancies. Every month there is a seminar for the gynecologists on gynecological psychosomatics. The department is also the clinical setting of the Institute for the Family and Sexological Sciences (30 h for all the students of the final year and one year for specialized training in family or marital therapy for psychologists-sexologists). During their clerkship in gynecology and obstetrics medical students take part in the weekly gynecological psychosomatic discussions.

## Other Activities

In the rehabilitation hospital of Pellenberg (University of Leuven), medical students and residents can observe various problems in consultative-liaison psychiatry:

(1) Diagnostic questions (mainly directed to the psychiatrist): these are questions concerning either possible psychological factors in somatic complaints (i.e. hysterical gait disturbances, psychogenic pain, psychogenic respiratory complaints), or the evaluation of psychiatric problems in somatically ill patients (i.e. a vital depression in a rheumatic patient, a confusional state in a postcoronary bypass patient). The diagnostic psychiatric evaluation consists of 1 or 2 interviews of 1 h; if necessary psychological testing is requested and finally it is completed with a report that includes a detailed diagnostic discussion and a therapeutic suggestion.

(2) Therapeutic questions (mainly directed to the psychologist): these are questions concerning psychological support of rehabilitation patients, pre- and postoperative patients, patients with relational or psychosocial difficulties, etc.

(3) Relaxation therapy: this treatment is frequently requested for patients with somatically unexplained or untreatable pains [56, 57], contractures, respiratory disturbances and postinfarction patients. After their stay at the hospital, patients who require further therapeutic aid are referred to another clinic (i.e. a mental health center) closer to their home. A limited number of outpatients are followed by the psychiatrist and the psychologist at Pellenberg.

(4) Questions concerning the 'psychological coaching' of the nursing staff (mainly done by the psychologist): the psychologist who assists the staff of the rheumatology and the rehabilitation sections is regularly asked for advice concerning attitude and relationship problems with 'difficult' patients. Problems concerning the relationship between the team members, or between the nursing staff and the medical staff, are also discussed.

## Perspectives of Consultation-Liaison Psychiatry

Although the gap between somatic and psychological or psychosocial thinking in medicine has been narrowed during the last 30 years, a genuine integrated approach to the patient remains rather difficult. The individualistic philosophy in our medical thinking and organization is the common denominator for the difficulties in reaching this synthetic approach to clinical problems. It starts in medical education, directed almost entirely to the growth of individual knowledge and skills. The future doctor is trained to obtain maximal skills to function as an individual helper to the patient as well as to take individual responsibility for his acts. In general, his teachers are highly specialized professionals, stressing their own individual viewpoints even on topics not belonging to their own area of experience. For the medical student the ideal doctor is an individual with a maximal professional knowledge and capacities to care for 'his' patient. Demonstrations of a real 'team' approach with shared tasks and responsibilities are unusual in classical medical education. Techniques of communicating with the patient have been introduced in the medical curriculum but communication between medical professionals of different specialties remains improvised and neglected. Communication with other health care professionals (psychologists, social workers, nurses, etc.) is not even taken into consideration. Thus the basic capacities of communication necessary to integrate the divergent views of somatic medicine, psychology and social science can hardly be achieved in the medical education. In Belgium, the typical medical graduate is an individual with respectable knowledge, devoted but rather possessive towards his patients. He respects but often does not understand the views of colleagues and other health professionals.

This individualistic attitude gets reinforcement by the organization of hospital medicine and the remuneration modalities of the health insurance system. Hospitals are organized as conglomerates of different departments, characterized by their specific ideology and technology. Differentiation is considered more important than integration. A person staying in a given department is labeled as a patient of that department or sometimes – when several doctors have their own divisions in a department – of a particular doctor. One can take the other doctor's advice but his own opinion remains preeminent towards the patient. There exist no departments of 'integrated' medicine, not even of 'psychosomatic' medicine. The achievement of some forms of integrated collaboration – such as the liaison psychiatry facility described above – depends entirely on the good will and initiatives of the doctors involved but finds no basis in the structural organization of the hospital.

These considerations may sound pessimistic for the future of consultative liaison psychiatry in Belgium. We feel it is necessary to present an honest and realistic view of the unfavorable background due to the official medical structure and organization. More optimistic elements can be detected since there is a steadily growing interest by doctors, mostly the young and idealistic, in psychological and psychosocial aspects in illness. This has initiated innovative educational formats for the introduction of psychological and psychosocial approaches in medical practice. It will also contribute to a slow but progressive elaboration of liaison psychiatry in Belgium!

## References

1   Dewachter, M.; Brosens, I.; Nijs, P.; Steeno, P.; Van Assche, A.; Vereecken, R.: Menselijke vruchtbaarheid en geboorteplanning. Het paar en zijn begeleidend team. (Elsevier Sequoia, Brussels 1976).

2   Dowiakowski, M.L. de; Luminet, D.: Etude psychosomatique de 32 cas d'infarctus du myocarde. Acta neurol. psychiat. belg. 69: 78–89 (1969).

3   Dumon, W.; Nijs, P.; Rouffa, L.; Steeno, O.: Donor insemination. A preliminary social and psychological report. Actes Colloque Internationale de Sexologie: Insemination artificielle et reproduction humaine, Leuven 1973, pp. 25–35.

4   Duret-Cosyns, S.; Luminet, D.: Les thérapies en médecine psychosomatique. Acta neurol. psychiat. belg. 69: 101–122 (1969).

5   Goldfarb, S.; Luminet, D.: Illustration de la relation objectale dans un cas d'ulcère de la cornée. Acta neurol. psychiat. belg. 69: 90–100 (1969).

6   Haber, M.; Luminet, D.: Experimental study of heart rate variability during studies on the psychophysiology of the cardio-pulmonary systems and attempt to obtain classical conditioning of heart rate by utilisation of unconditional stimuli belonging to the second system of signalisation; in Pierloot, Recent research in psychosomatics, pp. 254–258 (Karger, Basel 1970).

7   Haber, M.; Luminet, D.: Psychophysiologie de la respiration. III. Le souffle et le soupir. Revue Méd. psychosomat. 14: 137–150 (1972).

8   Hoornaert, F.; Pierloot, R.; Vertommen, H.: Blood pressure responses to stress in renal patients. Psychother. Psychosom. *17:* 178–190 (1969).

9   Hoornaert, F.; Pierloot, R.: The investment of paternal and maternal symbolism in the doctor image by non-patients. Medikon *5:* 33–40 (1976).

10  Hoornaert, F.; Pierloot, R.: Paternal and maternal symbolism in the parental images of psychosomatic and neurotic patients. J. psychosom. Res. *20:* 237–246 (1976).

11  Hoornaert, F.; Pierloot, R.: Transference aspects of doctor-patient relationship in psychosomatic patients. Br. J. med. Psychol. *49:* 261–266 (1976).

12  Luminet, D.: Psychothérapie brève de l'asthme bronchique. Acta neurol. psychiat. belg. *7:* 582–587 (1957).

13  Luminet, D.: Examen critique des modèles théoriques en recherche psychosomatique. Acta neurol. psychiat. belg. *4:* 417–489 (1959).

14  Luminet, D.: Les céphalalgies: point de vue psychosomatique. Bruxelles méd. *5:* 159–175 (1959).

15  Luminet, D.; Sloanaker, J.: Tentative expérimentale de conditionnement de la crise d'asthme bronchique et de son interruption chez l'homme. Revue Méd. psychosom. *3:* 225–249 (1962).

16  Luminet, D.; Feifer, T.; Van Reeth, P.C.: Le coronarien et son travail. Acta neurol. psychiat. belg. *69:* 69–77 (1969).

17  Luminet, D.: Etudes de psychophysiologie de la respiration. I. Suggestion et dysfonctionnement respiratoire. Acta neurol. psychiat. belg. *69:* 123–147 (1969).

18  Luminet, D.: Etudes de psychophysiologie de la respiration. II. Pavlov et Freud. Essai de synthèse. Acta neurol. psychiat. belg. *69:* 147–176 (1969).

19  Luminet, D.; Haber, M.: Les communications en psychophysiologie expérimentale chez l'homme. Revue Méd. psychosom. *13:* 391–407 (1971).

20  Luminet, D.: Le problème de l'investigation psychosomatique en gynécologie. Feuilles psychiat. Liège *8:* 27–32 (1975).

21  Luminet, D.: Nosographie psychanalytique et pathologie digestive. Acta gastroenter. belg. *38:* 403–409 (1975).

22  Luminet, D.; Defourny, M.; Hubin, P.: Alexithymia, 'pensée opératoire' and 'predisposition to coronopathy', pattern 'A' of Friedman and Rosenman. Psychother. Psychosom. *27:* 106–114 (1976/77).

23  Nijs, P.: Psychogener oder exogener Einfluss der Ovulationshemmer auf das Sexualverhalten und die Psychosexualität. Klinische Bemerkungen. J. neuro-visc. Relat., suppl. X, pp. 444–449 (1971).

24  Nijs, P.: Psychosomatische Aspekte der oralen Antikonzeption; in Burger-Prinz, Giese, Beiträge zur Sexualforschung, Heft 50 (Enke, Stuttgart 1972).

25  Nijs, P.: Psychodynamic aspects of oral contraception. Medikon *3:* 11–19 (1974).

26  Nijs, P.; Rouffa, L.: AID couples: psychological and psychopathological evaluation. Andrologia *7:* 187–194 (1975).

27  Nijs, P.: La pilule et la sexualité. Mythes et faits (Acco, Leuven 1975).

28  Nijs, P.: Aspects psychosomatiques de l'insémination artificielle; in Diererich, Pundel, Gynécologie psychosomatique et sexologie (European Press, Ghent 1976).

29  Nijs, P.; Rouffa, L.: AID couples: psychological and psychopathological evaluation; in Hirsch, Psychosomatic medicine in obstetrics and gynaecology, pp. 222–225 (Karger, Basel 1976).

30    Nijs, P.: Der Arzt und die kontrazeptive Beratung. Schriftenreihe BPA *4:* 51–53 (1977); Prakt. Arzt *22:* 3564–3570 (1977).

31    Nijs, P.; Hoppenbrouwers, L.: Adoption and AID couples. Psychosexual aspects. Fert. Steril. *28:* 370 (1977).

32    Nijs, P.: Psychological aspects of reversal of sterilization; in Brosens, Winston, Reversibility of female sterilization, pp. 167–174 (Academic Press/Grune & Stratton, New York 1978).

33    Nijs, P.: Arzt, Patient und Pille. Gedanken zur Medikation. Sexualmedizin *7:* 794–799 (1978).

34    Nijs, P.; Steeno, P.; Steppe, A.: Evaluation of AID donors: medical and psychological aspects. A preliminary report; in David, Price, Human artificial insemination and semen preservation, pp. 453–459 (Plenum Press, New York 1980).

35    Nijs, P.; Molinski, H.; Dmoch, W.; Höffken, K.-D.; Beusen, L.: Funktionelle Sexualstörungen, modifizierte Masters-Johnson Therapie. Inform. Arzt *9:* 74–75 (1981).

36    Nijs, P.: Fokussierende Sexualtherapie; in Vogt, Herms, Eicher, Praktische Sexualmedizin, pp. 225–230 (Medical Tribune, Wiesbaden 1981).

37    Nijs, P.: Psychological aspects of the pain experience; in Renaer, Chronic pelvic pain in women, pp. 24–31 (Springer, Berlin 1981).

38    Pierloot, R.: Aspects psychosomatiques de la médecine sociale et préventive. Scalpel *28:* 1–11 (1954).

39    Pierloot, R.: Les fondements de la conception psychosomatique dans la pratique médicale. Scalpel *19:* 1–15 (1956).

40    Pierloot, R.: Problèmes généraux de psychosomatique clinique (Nauwelaerts, Louvain/Béatrice, Paris 1956).

41    Pierloot, R.; Gelissen, L.; Reynders, M.: Psycho-social factors in industrial absenteeism by illness, in Advances in psychosomatic medicine, pp. 82–95 (Brunner, New York 1961).

42    Pierloot, R.: Phénomènes psychosomatiques et significations du corps pour la personne. Acta psychother. *9:* 295–303 (1961).

43    Pierloot, R.: Principes généraux de traitement en médecine psychosomatique. Acta neurol. psychiat. belg. *62:* 804–819 (1962).

44    Pierloot, R.; Boucquey, J.P.: L'anamnèse orientée dans le sens psychologique. Acta psychother. *11:* 445–463 (1963).

45    Pierloot, R.; Houben, M.E.: The scientific investigation of the therapeutic relationship; in Acta medica psychosomatica, pp. 44–49 (Settimane Psicosomatica Internazionale, Rome 1967).

46    Pierloot, R.: Collaboration hospitalière en médecine psychosomatique. Méd. Hyg. *26:* 134 (1968).

47    Pierloot, R.; Van Roy, J.: Asthma and aggression. J. psychosom. Res. *13:* 333–337 (1969).

48    Pierloot, R.: Recent research in psychosomatics (Karger, Basel 1970).

49    Pierloot, R.; De Bleeker, M.: Relationship patterns and their expression in the doctor-patient relation in asthmatics. Br. J. med. Psychol. *45:* 345–354 (1972).

50    Pierloot, R.: Psychiatric teaching to medical students in Belgium. Psychiat. Ann. *6:* 15–25 (1972).

51    Pierloot, R.; Hoornaert, F.: The image of the doctor in psychosomatic and psycho-

neurotic patients; in Antonelli, Therapy in psychosomatic medicine, I, pp. 163–177 (Pozzi, Rome 1975).

52   Pierloot, R.; Vinck, J.: A pragmatic approach to the concept of alexithymia. Psychother. Psychosom. *28:* 156–166 (1977).

53   Pierloot, R.; Hoornaert, F.: Parental symbolism in the doctor image of asthmatic patients. Psychother. Psychosom. *30:* 18–27 (1978).

54   Renaer, M.; Nijs, P.; Van Assche, A.; Vertommen, H.: Chronic pelvic pain without obvious pathology in women. Eur. J. Obstet. Gynec. reprod. Biol. *10:* 415 463 (1980).

55   Van Houdenhove, B.: Het gesprek met de psychosomatische patiënt. Tijdschr. Geneesk. *34:* 831–837 (1978).

56   Van Houdenhove, B.: Over de psychogene pijn. Tijdschr. Psychiat. *22:* 254–266 (1980).

57   Van Houdenhove, B.: Recente ontwikkelingen in de diagnostische classificatie van psychisch beïnvloede lichamelijke klachten. Tijdschr. Geneesk. *37:* 779–783 (1981).

R.A. Pierloot, MD, Professor of Psychiatry, Head of the Department of Psychiatry, University of Leuven, B–3000 Leuven (Belgium)

Adv. psychosom. Med., vol. 11, pp. 164–165 (Karger, Basel 1983)

# Consultation-Liaison Activities in West Germany: Introduction

*Hellmuth Freyberger, Karl Kohle, Hubert Speidel*

German departments of psychosomatics and psychotherapy generally represent divisions independent from psychiatry. Historically the 'psychosomatic movement' in the thirties was destroyed as the consequence of its psychoanalytic orientation under the Nazi regime. Psychoanalysts were so preoccupied with reestablishing their specific institutions that they did not have time for psychosomatic medicine. Concurrently German psychiatrists opposed the development of psychosomatic units until the beginning of the sixties. In this vacuum, four German internists and directors of university departments of medicine – *Paul Christian* (Heidelberg), *Arthur Jores* (Hamburg), *Walter Seitz* (Munich), *Thure von Uexküll* (Giessen, Ulm) – founded their own psychosomatic divisions. Thus a close relationship between psychosomatics and medicine has evolved.

The combination of internist and psychosomaticist is a frequent one in the present generation of German psychosomaticists. Independent psychosomatic divisions exist in the majority of the 22 German medical schools. Traditional psychiatric patients, e.g. organic brain syndrome, endogenous depression, schizophrenia, alcoholism, drug dependence and suicidal problems, are not seen by psychosomaticists but by the psychiatrists. The psychosomaticist examines and treats the following two patient groups: (1) patients who are suffering from so-called psychosomatic disorders; (2) patients who are suffering from so-called primary organic diseases who show present conflict situations and/or marked secondary psychic alterations. The majority of the German psychosomaticists are psychoanalytically oriented. Nevertheless, behavioral therapists are also available.

The psychosomatic and psychotherapy divisions are organized to include the following three sections: (1) the outpatient clinic as an entry point to patient care; (2) the 'Innere Ambulanz', i.e. the consultation-liaison activities to the other clinical departments outside of psychiatry and psychosomatics, and (3) dedicated inpatient unit for psychosomatic patients.

Following a drastic reform of the medical curriculum in the early sixties, psychosomatics and psychotherapy are taught to medical students. Three didactic strategies are utilized [*Meyer*, 1979]: didactic lectures, interviewing skills experience, and self-awareness experiences such as Balint groups comprised of students. This chapter will present current activities in consultation-liaison at Ulm, Hamburg and Hannover.

*Reference*

Meyer, A.E.: German developments in teaching psychosomatics and psychotherapy to medical students. Psychother. Psychosom. *31:* 75–80 (1979).

H. Freyberger, MD, Professor of Psychosomatics, Hannover Medical School, Karl-Wiechert-Allee 9, D–3000 Hannover 61 (FRG)

Adv. psychosom. Med., vol. 11, pp. 166–175 (Karger, Basel 1983)

# Clinical and Educational Activities of a Psychosomatic Division

*Hellmuth Freyberger, Jutta Nordmeyer, Hans-Werner Künsebeck,*
*Wolfgang Lempa, Hans-Jürgen Avenarius, Walter Wellmann,*
*Reinhard Liedtke, Rolf Schöl*

Department of Psychosomatics, Hannover Medical School, Hannover, FRG

The Hannover Medical School, opened in 1964, utilizes broad inter-disciplinary cooperation. This interdisciplinary approach fosters positive attitudes towards psychosomatics and psychotherapy. In Hannover, the Department of Psychosomatics has existed since 1975. The Hannover section includes a director and 8 full-time co-workers (2 internists, 2 psychiatrists and 4 psychologists), 6 of which are psychoanalytically trained and 1 is undergoing psychoanalytical training. Another co-worker is a psychologist and behavioral therapist who is responsible for directing research.

## Clinical Activities

In Hannover, the two main consultation-liaison activities are the following: (1) the psychosomatic inpatient ward, and (2) the 'Innere Ambulanz' which is the psychosomatic consultation division.

### Inpatient Ward

The Hannover psychosomatic inpatient ward located within the general hospital comprises 14 beds. The patients treated there are either directly transferred from the medical wards or come from our outpatient clinic. The main criteria for admission is the patient's ability to utilize the psychoanalytically oriented group psychotherapy, our chief therapeutic strategy that lasts 2 months. The psychologically minded patients with anorexia nervosa, obesity, labile essential hypertension, bronchial asthma, selected cases of ulcerative colitis and Crohn's disease as well as certain functional somatic disorders (especially cardiac neuroses) are most suitable. Besides psychoanalytically oriented group psychotherapy, other therapeutic activities such as individual talks, creative activities, gymnastics, relaxation, interaction exercises and rhythmics are performed by the nursing staff.

The goal of this inpatient ward psychotherapy is the intensifying of the patient's perception of his interpersonal conflicts and how they use their psychic and somatic symptomatology to mask intrapsychic conflicts. If the patients succeed in developing increased problem consciousness, then, frequently they not only obtain reduction of their psychic suffering but also increasing relief from somatic symptoms. Patients then can better cope with reality demands and frequently continue the psychoanalytic group therapy on an outpatient basis.

Besides these effective group experiences and the concurrent therapeutic procedures performed by nurses, the psychosomatic inpatient ward includes the following two consultation-liaison activities: (1) the close cooperation of the psychosomaticists with other doctors during the selection and transfer of patients to our psychosomatic ward as well as the internists consultative functions for medical problems during mutual rounds which include internists, psychosomaticists and nurses, and (2) the regular participation of students as well as guest doctors and nurses in certain inpatient ward processes for the purpose of teaching.

### Settings Outside the Psychosomatic Unit

We try to separate the psychosomatic problems in inpatients (the 'Innere Ambulanz') from those of the 'Outpatient Clinic' ('Äussere Ambulanz'). Two broad patient groups emerge regarding the type of treatment received. First, outpatients who suffer from psychosomatic disorders and show some psychological motivation and average introspective ability independently seek out our outpatient clinic. This patient group represents the bulk of our group psychotherapy patients. Second, on the medical wards there are patients suffering from psychosomatic disorders or primary organic diseases who show distinct conflict situations and/or secondary psychic alterations (particularly states of hopelessness). These patients usually have limited introspective ability and very low motivation for psychodynamic interviews and psychotherapy. Nevertheless, these patients are transferred to us by the clinicomedical colleagues and treated initially by supportive psychotherapy (including cautious confrontations and surface interpretations). Innovative use of students allows sufficient personnel to deliver care.

Patients with little insight who possess psychological conflicts are rarely treated with insight oriented psychological strategies. Furthermore, a relatively small number of psychodynamically oriented psychotherapists are available for these inpatients. This limited availability results from the limited motivation of trained psychotherapists to treat these inpatients by supportive techniques. Many psychodynamically oriented psychotherapists consider medical inpatients too 'unyielding' and therefore not 'sufficiently interesting' for psychotherapeutic work. The countertransference reactions provoked in medical inpatients may further discourage the therapist. These reactions may be characterized by feelings of boredom and exhaustion; the psychotherapist's feeling of powerlessness and the connected narcissistic insult as the consequence of his threatening failure also make the work with these patients difficult.

Since supportive psychotherapy is a less complex procedure and the treatment of choice for these medical inpatients, we decided that student auxiliary therapists could be suitable therapists for medical inpatient care. This model began in November 1978, and has developed into an empirical study supported by the Volkswagen Foundation. To select the student auxiliary therapists, we accepted every student interested in serving a 4- to 5-month internship rotation. Thus, 80 students have worked as auxiliary therapists.

### The Student Auxiliary Therapist

To clarify the student's work, we will outline the following two inpatient consultation-liaison activities.

#### Initial Interview

The goal of the patient-oriented consultation via initial interviews is to assess the patient's motivation to understand his problem and the feasibility of subsequent psychotherapeutic treatment. These student interviews promote the interdisciplinary oriented cooperation with the doctors and nurses. This cooperation includes the following: (1) if the doctors and nurses cannot solve the patient's problems by somatic means the care givers will become more acquainted with the patient's emotional status; (2) the psychotherapy adds to the somatic treatments, and (3) the introduction of the psychotherapy promotes regular meetings of the individual student with that doctor and nurse who are primarily responsible for the patient.

The student auxiliary therapists' effectiveness can be achieved only if the doctors and nurses who work in the inpatient wards are open-minded

*Table I.* Medical diagnoses in so-called psychosomatic (first group)[1] and so-called primary organically ill patients (second group)

| Diagnoses | n | % | |
|---|---|---|---|
| *First group* | | | |
| Crohn's disease | 25 | 13.1 | |
| Anorexia nervosa | 18 | 9.4 | |
| Ulcerative colitis | 17 | 8.9 | |
| Generalized functional disorders | 16 | 8.4 | |
| Bronchial asthma | 15 | 7.8 | |
| Irritable bowel syndrome | 10 | 5.2 | |
| Chronic factious disorders with physical symptoms | 7 | 3.7 | |
| Sudden deafness | 7 | 3.7 | |
| Obesity | 6 | 3.1 | 74.3% |
| Duodenal ulcer | 6 | 3.1 | |
| Osphyalgia | 5 | 2.6 | |
| Nonorganic 'rheumatism' of soft tissue | 3 | 1.6 | |
| Hyperventilation tetany | 2 | 1.1 | |
| Torticollis | 2 | 1.1 | |
| Labile essential hypertension | 1 | 0.5 | |
| Cardiac neurosis | 1 | 0.5 | |
| Impotentia | 1 | 0.5 | |
| *Second group* | | | |
| Accident service | 13 | 6.8 | |
| End-stage renal failure | 8 | 4.2 | |
| Cancer[2] | 5 | 2.6 | |
| Rheumatoid arthritis | 4 | 2.1 | |
| Chronic pancreatitis | 3 | 1.6 | |
| Epilepsy | 3 | 1.6 | |
| Postoperative states | 3 | 1.6 | 25.7% |
| Chronic bronchitis | 2 | 1.1 | |
| Diabetes mellitus | 2 | 1.1 | |
| Organic angina pectoris | 1 | 0.5 | |
| Fixed essential hypertension | 1 | 0.5 | |
| Bechterew's disease | 1 | 0.5 | |
| Bone marrow depression | 1 | 0.5 | |
| Dermatomyositis | 1 | 0.5 | |
| Liver transplant | 1 | 0.5 | |
| Total | 191 | 100 | |

[1] Patients suffering from essential hypertension are particularly examined by a separate group of behavioral therapists.

[2] A separate consultation liaison group occurs in cancer patients supplementary being psychotherapeutically treated; furthermore, concerning the latter patients hospital clergymen with both clinical and pastoral training are also very active.

*Table II.* Patient distributions concerning age and sex

| Age | Female | Male | Total |
|---|---|---|---|
| 20 | 21 | 11 | 32 |
| 21–30 | 30 | 24 | 54 |
| 31–40 | 22 | 11 | 33 |
| 41–50 | 24 | 13 | 37 |
| 51–60 | 15 | 10 | 25 |
| 61–70 | 2 | 6 | 8 |
| 71 | 2 | 0 | 2 |
| | 116 | 75 | 191 |
| | (61%) | (39%) | (100%) |

with regard to psychosomatics and psychotherapy, and the students are supervised daily in a group format of 8 students on their individual psychotherapy.

### Indications for Psychotherapy

The patients who are treated by professional therapists in our psychosomatic inpatient ward with psychoanalytically oriented techniques initially show more introspective ability in contrast to those patients who have the same medical diagnoses but stay in the clinicomedical inpatient wards and are treated by the students. Here, the conflict working procedure in the sense of psychoanalytically oriented group psychotherapy cannot be applied, at least not immediately, but supportive psychotherapy (including cautious confrontations and surface interpretations) does.

The medical diagnoses of those 59 inpatients who are suffering from primary organic diseases who also demonstrate psychological conflicts and/or marked secondary psychic alterations are shown in table I. The distribution with regard to our psychosomatic and primary organically ill patients, concerning their age and sex are presented in table II.

Very few patients on medical services can utilize insight oriented depth psychotherapy. A cohort was studied in which 178 introductory psychodynamic interviews were performed by senior faculty members. Supportive psychotherapy (including cautious confrontations and surface interpretations) was indicated in 157 patients (table III).

On the basis of these findings it is evident that there were no reasons to refer patients to our psychosomatic inpatient ward or use psychoanalyti-

*Table III.* Indications with regard to psychotherapy

|  | n | % |
| --- | --- | --- |
| Indication concerning psychosomatic inpatient ward | – | – |
| Indication concerning psychoanalytically orientated techniques on an outpatient basis | – | – |
| Indication concerning supportive psychotherapy | 157 | 88 |
| No indication concerning supportive psychotherapy | 21 | 12 |
|  | 178 | 100 |

cally oriented techniques on an outpatient basis. In the further 21 cases, the supportive psychotherapeutic indication did not occur. In spite of recommendation for supportive psychotherapy, this treatment rarely took place because of a lack of motivation, or because of sudden deterioration in their physical condition. From these findings there is clear support to document the reduced introspective ability and low motivation for dynamic psychotherapy in such medical inpatients.

*Supportive Psychotherapy*

Supportive psychotherapy can begin following the diagnostic interview as well as consensual agreement by the primary physician. The treatment relationship allows a stable oral-narcissistic object relationship. The three phases emerge: (1) Initial ventilation of hypochondriacal concerns characterizes the patient's early verbalizations. This ventilation promotes the less differentiated patient 'to speak about himself' and allow marked emotional relief. (2) The second step includes the encouragement of the patient to verbalize more differentiated self-reflections and feelings, particularly feelings of narcissistic insult, depression and frustration-aggression. Cautious confrontations by the student may be utilized. (3) If more differentiated verbalizations are manifest, we are able to superficially deal with the patient's present conflict situations and/or psychological problems in connection with his disease.

The inclusion of relatives for the purpose of couple interviews or family therapy occurs in two thirds of the patients. This format may be arranged directly following the psychodynamic interviews or later on in the course of the treatment. The goals for our family therapy include an opportunity for (1) relatives to become familiar with our psychotherapeutic interest; (2) the patient to perceive in a more differentiated way his marital and family interactions; (3) the therapist to observe the patient's interactions with his family.

The supportive psychotherapeutic effects in the psychosomatic inpatients and the primary organically ill patients foster emotional security and allow psychic relief due to the stable student-patient relationship. Frequently this emotional security may include increased self-reflection and conflict consciousness which foster the indication for continuing dynamic psychotherapy. 4–5 treatment hours per patient is the most common frequency. Half of all patients utilized seven treatments or less while 73.1% used less than 14 sessions.

### Aftercare

Follow-up treatment is necessary for both psychological and somatic problems. This is achieved by collaboration with the primary physician and psychosomaticist. Thus, follow-up 'psychosomatic' care is frequent. Agreements must exist between the primary medical staff and the psychosomaticist to arrange both somatic and psychological care.

### Psychosomatic Inpatient Care

We may refer a patient to our psychosomatic inpatient ward if increased self-reflection ability and conflict awareness, achieved first by supportive psychotherapy, allows utilization of dynamically oriented psychotherapy. This necessitates that the psychosomatic patient becomes a psychoneurotic patient. In other cases, those patients who were successfully treated by supportive psychotherapy often do not require continuing psychotherapy. For others it is often necessary to have a continuation of the supportive psychotherapy in the outpatient setting following the inpatient stay in the medical ward. In Hannover, this outpatient psychotherapy is performed by supervised student auxiliary therapists. Following this supportive psychotherapy, a number of those patients are suitable for admission to our psychosomatic inpatient ward.

Following long-term supportive psychotherapy, it also may emerge that the patient's psychic disorders are too serious with regard to a successful psychotherapeutic work in our psychosomatic inpatient ward. In this case, the transfer to a psychosomatic psychotherapeutic special hospital is necessary.

## Team-Oriented Activity

The team-oriented activity corresponds to the need of certain medical staff, both doctors and nurses, for team advice about the psychological issues of their patients. In this particular case, our supervision group came to an agreement that the student alone or together with the professional psychosomaticist should give the advice. We have established group meetings with nurses in units dedicated to dialysis, general and renal transplantation surgery, oncology, gastroenterology, open heart surgery and accident surgery. These specially scheduled conferences are independent from the regular meetings of the individual student with the doctor and nurse responsible for an individual patient. The topics of the specially scheduled conferences include *both* advice concerning the psychological treatment of problem in-patients *and* investigation of tensions between the nurses and doctors. Two chief difficulties in arranging these conferences exist: (1) due to our training system there is high movement of the professionals from one ward to another. Therefore, continuous group work with a stable group membership is complicated. (2) For nurses and doctors to carefully reflect about their own perceptions vis-à-vis their patients may be subjectively painful and difficult. These difficulties are the consequence of the fact that in Germany the nurses and doctors of the present generation were minimally trained about the psychological aspects of their patients.

## Reactions of the Student Therapists

The educational program in which the student therapists participate has augmented their introspective capacity. Concurrently they have responded to their clinical responsibilities with marked enthusiasm. In our view, the main reason for this enhanced introspective ability and enthusiasm is that the students are able to experience a clinical relationship with the same patient. In addition, their own responsibility on the medical wards and close cooperation with the primary doctors and nurses gives them increased self-esteem. As the consequence of this experience, the students were able to quickly overcome anxiety about whether they would be 'good enough' as a therapist. According to this experience, there exists no more optimal education than the student's undertaking clinical responsibility for a patient. It is our impression that the psychotherapeutic effectiveness of the students is at least the same, even if higher, than that of the professional psychotherapists.

The excellent psychotherapeutic results may be due to the following four issues: (1) the students are able to optimally develop with the patient a 'symbiosis for a short time' and not play a 'neutral' role; (2) the students are more 'naive' and enthusiastic; (3) the students are better able to tolerate the countertransference reaction vis-à-vis the patient; (4) the students are at the lower end of the medical status hierarchy and, therefore, the social distance to the patient is less in comparison with the doctors group. This also fosters a more stable student-patient relationship.

### Consultative Psychiatry versus Liaison Medicine

Our model in Hannover is closer to a consultative model. The students are chiefly based in the Department of Psychosomatics and, hence, they perform their tasks on medical units. Therefore, the students are not a 'solid' and 'stable' part of a clinicomedical department, team or unit as in a 'pure' liaison setting. However, due to the many students working as auxiliary therapists on medical units, psychosomatics has high visibility in Hannover. Thus, our model is on the continuum from consultative psychiatry to liaison medicine. In fact, the students are fully accepted as direct cooperating partners by the doctors and nurses all the time they are engaged in the longitudinal process of supportive psychotherapy within the medical wards. Furthermore, the students are included at case conferences and in important decision discussions which concern their patients. Finally, the students are engaged in arranging both the regular meetings and specialty conferences with the doctors and nurses on the wards.

Due to our staff limitations, we are not able to give continuous advice throughout the clinicomedical wards and some inpatients do not experience the advantage of psychologicomedical examinations and needed psychotherapies. But for the purpose of achieving the 'liaison' principle one serious problem occurs. If we intend to arrange successful liaison services, we can achieve it in some selected wards only. We feel it is more advantageous to offer psychosomatics to the whole hospital and cooperate in selected cases than concentrate on a single ward. In our view the main advantage of this approach is to allow continuous psychotherapy with individual patients staying in various wards. On this basis, a disproportionately larger number of doctors and nurses may simultaneously participate in our procedures even if this cooperation is not so close as in the case of the relatively more intensively oriented 'liaison' approach.

Thus, the student auxiliary therapist activities in our 'Innere Ambulanz' represent an optimal consultation liaison model because of the following three features: (1) Their clinical services within the medical inpatient settings does not create a financial burden; (2) patients are treated who need psychotherapy but until now have not received it, and (3) the students are trained in a psychotherapy which will later benefit the general population.

## Research

Our research activities with regard to the student auxiliary therapists activities includes the following five areas: (1) The documentation of our psychosomatico-psychotherapeutic inpatient care model. (2) Empirical examination of the quantitative needs for the supplementary psychosomatico-psychotherapeutic inpatient care within the medical units. (3) The evaluation of the patients' psychotherapy. This evaluation starts from the obvious psychologicomedical differences in patients suffering from ulcerative colitis and Crohn's disease. On this basis, the effectiveness of the supportive psychotherapy should be proven empirically in these two inpatient groups (under inclusion of control groups), particularly also on the basis of their subsequent outpatient psychotherapy setting including the evaluation of the cost-effectiveness effects due to psychotherapeutic procedures. On the other hand, this evaluation of psychotherapy concerns the other inpatient groups who are not only tested by student auxiliary therapists but also by psychodynamically oriented psychotherapists for the purpose of clarification concerning the clinically relevant effectivity problem of 'professional therapists versus lay therapists'. (4) The evaluation of the reactions of the auxiliary therapist function on the students. (5) The further basic improvements with regard to the training model of the student auxiliary therapists.

H. Freyberger, MD, Professor of Psychosomatics, Hannover Medical School, Karl-Wiechert-Allee 9, D–3000 Hannover 61 (FRG)

Adv. psychosom. Med., vol. 11, pp. 176–190 (Karger, Basel 1983)

# The Psychosomatic Ward

*Karl Köhle*

Department of Psychosomatic Medicine, University of Ulm, FRG

## Goals

Ulm University was founded as a 'reform university' in 1967. It is a small university with only two faculties, medicine and science. In 1981 the medical faculty had a total of 1,750 students.

The reform was aimed at several goals. In medicine, clinically oriented research and interdisciplinary cooperation in patient care were to be encouraged. The reorganization of clinical work into a departmental system was a new idea in the Federal Republic of Germany at the time and was hoped to counteract a splitting up of medicine into various subdisciplines. Psychosomatic medicine was to represent a strong point in research and patient care; its function was to add the psychosocial dimension to the biological approach in medicine. The Department of Internal Medicine and Psychosomatics was part of the Centre for Internal Medicine. The department's first head, *Thure von Uexküll* (1967–1976) also held one of the chairs for internal medicine. It was one of the jobs of the department to participate fully in the provision of general medical care. At the same time it was to introduce and set up a biopsychosocial approach in the centre as a whole. Apart from the head of department, the departmental staff included one senior doctor, five residents, two psychologists and a social worker. The medical members of staff had either already specialized or were still specializing in internal medicine. The majority was also in psychoanalytic training. On the whole, the psychodynamic approach dominated work in the department, although one psychologist was behaviourally oriented.

Three members of staff were in charge of general medical wards. There they were supposed to realize a holistic psychosomatic approach in an exemplary fashion. Two senior members of staff, who were more advanced in their psychotherapeutic training, provided a liaison service and gave support to colleagues on other wards, if problems arose in connection with psychosocial aspects. Consultation was doctor- or team-oriented.

The department also set up a small psychosomatic outpatient service and a special outpatient service for patients suffering from high blood pressure. A research laboratory was attached to the latter.

Work at the department was supported by another independent university department, the Department of Psychotherapy, which provided further training courses for members of staff.

The psychosomatic approach was also integrated into the teaching of medical students. Practical work in psychosomatic medicine was combined with practical work in internal medicine. One of its main teaching aims is to familiarize students with the technique of the clinical interview as described by *Morgan and Engel* [1969].

### Experiences Made during the First 5 Years (1967–1972)

In 1972 we undertook a first 'balancing of the books' [*von Uexküll*, 1973; *Karstens*, 1973; *Schüffel*, 1973; *Rotmann*, 1973; *Köhle* et al., 1973]. There were gratifying signs of cooperation in teaching and research, here especially with the oncologists. Success in the field of patient care was only very modest, however. We had to acknowledge that we had not succeeded in gaining any crucial influence in patient care as was provided by the Centre for Internal Medicine. The biological approach still dominated. Individual physicians might have paid more attention to psychosocial factors than their colleagues at traditional internal clinics, but on the whole, we had not succeeded in integrating psychosomatic medicine, according to its scientific standing, into general patient care. This was also true of our own work as ward doctors; external conditions were not right, e.g. it was not possible to modify working processes on the wards according to the requirements of the psychosomatic approach.

Looking back today, I would say that we greatly underestimated the conflicts brought about by the attempt to change the traditional system of internal medical care in such a way as to take the psychosocial dimension into account systematically. Considerable organizational changes are necessary, if such an expansion of the theory is to be put into practice; such changes can meet with strong opposition which we were not prepared for.

Trying to make conceptual changes without changing external conditions meant we were asking too much even of our motivated colleagues among the internal specialists.

Our own situation as 'psychosomaticists' in internal medicine also had to remain unsatisfactory. We had no distinct area in which to try out this combination of somatic and psychosocial approaches. Thus the development of a specific identity as 'psychosomaticists' remained a problem for us.

### The Internal-Psychosomatic Ward (1972–1979)

This was the situation when, in 1972, we were given the opportunity to take over a general medical ward with 15 beds. Here we could reorganize working structures according to our own ideas.

One of the prerequisites for the successful integration of the psychosomatic approach into work on a hospital ward is a certain flexibility in the social field. The patient must be able to enter into relationships with doctors and nurses depending on his particular needs and conflicts. Ward staff must be given the opportunity to reflect on these relationships and to contribute the outcome of these reflections to the diagnostic and the therapeutic process. This is possible only where ward staff are willing to react to the individual patient and be moved by him – rather like the sounding box of a musical instrument. By reflecting on their co-movements they should try to perceive the impulses emanating from the patient and to understand them. Impulses emanating from members of staff might have their origin in an attitude of resistance towards a particular patient for example. As these could prevent the patient from reenacting his problems, they ought to be laid open to reflection as well.

A ward which has been reorganized successfully according to such principles has several advantages over the mere addition of psychotherapeutic modalities to medical treatment. Diagnosis and therapy take place in a milieu which has been modelled carefully on one concept. This milieu offers the patient the cognitive and emotional security he needs to enter into a working relationship with the doctor. The perceptions of individual team members add up to one more complete picture of the patient. The various therapeutic approaches can be coordinated within this conceptual framework. Information, which team members have received from patients, is more easily exchanged. Everyone is working in the same set-up, which in our case was created to suit the psychodynamic outlook we had chosen.

Diagnosis and therapy can benefit from relationships set up in the medical treatment situation. We assume that in the here and now of interactions with members of staff the patient presents his most important problems. These interactive problems are the focus of discussions at ward staff meetings. Thus, while an understanding of the patient's particular problems is gained, members of staff are given emotional support at the same time.

The following points ought to be considered in the attempt to integrate the psychosomatic approach into patient care.

(1) A *theoretical concept* ought to be at the base of such an attempt. This enables one to work on and gain an insight into the patient's intrapsychic processes as well as interactive processes taking place between the patient and team members. We adopted the psychoanalytic approach for this purpose.

(2) *Further training* of all involved should also be based on this concept. Doctors on our ward were undergoing postgraduate training in internal medicine and psychoanalysis; for nurses we introduced a 1-year fulltime course in 'psychosomatic medicine/patient-centered care' [*Köhle* et al., 1980].

(3) *Work* on the ward ought to be *organized* in such a way as to intensify relations between patients and members of staff. Exchange of information within the team ought to be encouraged. Doctors and nurses ought to receive sufficient emotional support in stressful situations which arise with an intensified contact with patients.

It was our *goal* to give *equal attention to somatic and psychosocial aspects in the diagnosis and therapy of every patient* from the day of his admission. Chosing this ward for our project we were able to investigate how far it is possible to modify the existing system of medical care towards a more patient-centered one. In other words, is it possible to 'loosen the tension between the poles of the individual vs. medical action within a bureaucratic organisation. . .' [*Raspe*, 1979].

Admission to this ward was by allocation through the reception at the Centre for Internal Medicine. This procedure was the same for all hospital departments.

The analysis of 998 instances of patients staying on the ward during a period of 3½ years (from 1975 to 1978) showed the following distribution. In 80% of the patients organic illness prevailed; approximately 20% of patients had functional disorders or 'psychosomatic illnesses' in the classical sense. 40% suffered from diseases of the circulatory system or the respiratory organs; 20% had cancer. 36% of the patients were classed by us as 'terminally ill' (criteria were: average period they had left to live $\leq 2$

*Table I.* The concepts of the full-time training course for nurses

| Behaviour training: patient-oriented nursing | Training in improving nursing organization | Psychosomatic theory |
|---|---|---|
| Interview training | team work on the ward | workshop teaching: |
| Nursing supervision | psychoanalytic experiential group | medical psychology and sociology |
| 'Balint groups' | systems of nursing organization | theory of neuroses and psychosomatic diseases |
| Psychoanalytic experiential group | information systems | psychiatry supportive psychotherapy social psychology and sociology of medical institutions |

years or/and risk of dying within the next 3 months $\geq 30\%$). Mortality rate on the ward was 10%.

The mean age of patients was 49.9 years; mean duration of stay during those 3½ years oscillated between 17.9 and 22.0 days; 50% of the patients stayed no longer than 14 days.

It was the goal of patient care reorganization to build a strong foundation for further and more specific psychotherapeutic measures. We replaced the traditional system of splitting up nursing into different functions by a system in which each nurse had full responsibility for several patients. This was to create and maintain a certain amount of continuity in the relationship. Numbers in the team were complemented by a psychosomatically trained nurse, who had a supervisory position and took on particular jobs in patient care. The support and cooperation of the Centre's head nursing staff made these changes a success.

The fact that we were working as a team (two ward doctors, one student doctor, six nurses, two student nurses and – on a parttime basis – a social worker, a psychologist and a hospital chaplain) required the laying-down of competencies and individual functions.

In order to improve cooperation between the various professional groups, it was essential to improve the postgraduate courses offered to nurses. Since 1975 we have been holding fulltime 1-year courses in 'patient-centered care/psychosomatic medicine'. Eight nurses can take part; during the first year also all the nurses working on the ward took the opportunity. During the year, work on the ward alternates with study periods in a 3-week cycle.

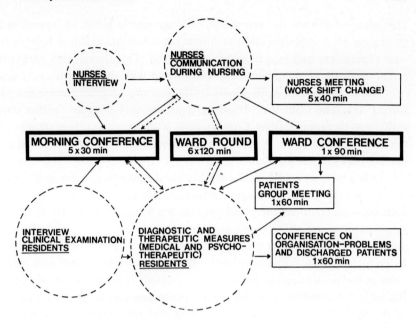

*Fig. 1.* Organization of the routine work on the ward.

More important than the acquisition of factual knowledge is the training in new behaviour patterns. Nurses practise interview and conversation techniques, first of all in role play, then under the supervision of the teaching nurse and finally in interactions with patients. These are videotaped (table I) and give an impression of the seminars and practical work offered.

Figure 1 illustrates the organization of work on the ward. Upon admission the patient is greeted by the nurse in charge. She conducts the *initial interview,* in which she tries to give the patient the impression of being welcome and that he has come to a place where he will be looked after. She is to attend to his needs personally in this often strange and worrying environment. During this interview she is particularly interested in the patient's own perception of his illness, in the kind and the extent of help he requires, in his subjective ideas about the nature and the consequences of his illness, in the expectations he has with regard to his stay in hospital, in his social situation and the conditions surrounding the onset of his illness. The nurse will use the information she has gained to formulate a *nursing diagnosis* and to draw up a *nursing plan.*

In a clinical interview [*Morgan and Engel,* 1969], which follows, the physician establishes the *anamnesis*. The patient is given an opportunity to present his complaints and the course his illness has taken in light of his own experiences and in a biographical context. The doctor pays particular attention to the development of a relationship with the patient.

Nurse and doctor both report to the *morning staff conference* the following day. The team then draws up a preliminary plan for further diagnostic and therapeutic steps. Competencies with regard to this particular patient are also laid down. A *list of medical problems* [*Weed*, 1971] as well as a *nursing plan* are put on file.

Other meetings, such as the weekly *ward conference*, serve as a forum, where information is exchanged, misunderstandings and emotional problems between team members and patients are worked on. We try to discuss in an exemplary fashion those problems, which a member of staff has in dealing with a particular patient. Observations and experiences made by individuals usually supplement each other; gaps are thus filled and distortions in the perceptions of individuals corrected. A better understanding of the patient is reached. The therapeutic procedure can be discussed in light of the patient's potential for development and with regard to the possible problems of individual team members. We also try to cope with the emotional strain that team members generally experience when working with patients who are seriously ill.

The extent of the strain showed up in the analysis of minutes which had been taken at 108 conferences from 1972 to 1978. During the first years the problems discussed mostly concerned patients with oncological illness; death and dying were the major issues. Problems of younger patients were by far overrepresented and perceived as particularly distressing. Only later on in the history of the ward did other questions come to be discussed as well, such as questions concerning the clarification of conflicts arising between team members and 'psychosomatic' patients. This development probably corresponds to the development of an ability to cope with the threat of experiencing loss, to cope with one's own anxieties and with mourning [*Gaus* et al., 1980].

We were particularly interested in changing the *ward round* in accordance with our goals. We tried to keep the situation at the bedside free (as much as possible) for a conversation between doctor and patient and for the medical examination. In order to do this, we split off all other functions of the visit. The discussion of test results and exchange of information between team members now takes place outside the patient's room prior to the visit. The visit is followed by a post-visit discussion of the conversation which has taken place between doctor and patient. Here further interventive steps are also considered. During the ward visit the patient should be given a chance to ask questions and to speak freely about his expectations. He should be able to take an active part in structuring the course of the conversation and should be encouraged to get involved in the diagnostic and therapeutic processes. The patient ought to be give adequate information about his situation. Such information must be given in comprehensible form. Interest shown by the doctor can have a stabilizing effect on the regulation of self-esteem and the ego functions. It is easier for the patient to orient himself in his situation if he is given information, which then has a supportive and an encouraging effect.

Many patients can be helped greatly in the process of *working through* the psychosocial implications of their *illness* by the ward round visit. *Problems in illness behaviour* can be mentioned and quite often be worked on in the immediate context. If the doctor succeeds in reaching the patient in his state of fear, depression or emotional withdrawal, in his anger or frustration about medicine or individual doctors, this might trigger off processes which can be taken up at further visits. The patient is given the chance to work on problems which have arisen in connection with his present condition. The *process of mourning* in seriously ill patients can especially be backed up in this way, in the context of medical care. In general, it is easier for the doctor, who normally examines and treats the patient, to give comfort and support than for a consultant, who is called in to deal with a 'psychological problem'.

The visit can also be used for *psychotherapeutic interventions* aimed at factors which have a pathogenetic effect. These possibilities of the ward round resemble those ideas developed by *Balint and Norell* [1973] in their concept of 'general practice psychotherapy'. The doctor can point out connections between the appearance of a complaint and emotional or situational causal factors and possibly motivate the patient to undergo psychotherapeutic treatment. This is facilitated by the fact that the patient's complaint and symptoms are attended to during the ward round visit. These are taken even more seriously, if put in a wider context.

The visit of the head of department was also modified according to our principles [*von Uexküll*, 1977; *Westphale and Köhle*, 1982]. Apart from performing supervisory functions the head of department also tries to keep the bedside situation free for conversations with the patient. An empirical investigation showed that this goal was largely attained.

It should be pointed out, that patients, who are seriously ill, are offered longer and more intensive conversations with a doctor or nurse in charge or – if indicated – formal psychotherapeutic sessions. It seems particularly important to us to keep the next-of-kin informed about diagnostic and, possibly also, therapeutic measures.

### Empirical Investigation of Effected Changes

With the help of tape recordings of ward round visits we examined the following question: had we succeeded in improving the physicians' speech behaviour and to what extent had it changed? We investigated the development of patient-centered attitudes in nurses, who were on the postgraduate course. We also looked at the development of emotional strain as the course progressed. Our data source was tape recordings made at 'Balint group' meetings which took place during the course.

The literature reports defects in the communicative behaviour of doctors on traditional hospital wards. In investigating visit contact, we were concerned with the question to what degree these defects had been eliminated. Had we institutionalized the necessary conditions for a true dialogue between doctor and patient?

The results are based on 615 visits. These were the first 5 visits made to 123 patients; these visits were made by 9 different doctors during 3½ years.

The results are compared with results obtained by similar methods at various 'Kreiskrankenhäuser' (county hospitals) in Baden-Württemberg and Hesse [Marburg studies: *Begemann-Deppe*, 1978; *Raspe*, 1979, 1982; *Raspe and Nordmeyer*, 1981; *Siegrist*, 1976, 1978], on a medical ward of a Hamburg hospital [*Jährig and Koch*, 1982; *Safian* et al., 1982] and at a rheumatism clinic [*Nordmeyer*, 1982]. This was not supposed to be a quantitative comparison; we were concerned with the question, whether the average present state can be changed with reasonable effort. If it can be changed, to what extent can it be changed? We have in the meantime made a systematic comparison between the wards at Ulm and Hamburg, for which patient samples were matched [*Safian* et al., 1982]. We examined the following points.

(1) Had *visit duration increased* by an extent which allowed for the development of a true relationship between doctor and patient?

(2) Did conversation at the bedside concentrate on a *dialogue* between doctor and patient?

(3) Was *participation evenly balanced* between doctor and patient?

(4) Had the *offer of information* been improved quantitatively and qualitatively?

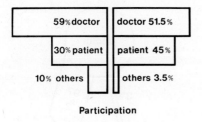

Participation

*Fig. 2.* Distribution of participation in conversation during rounds (%).

(5) Was the patient given greater opportunity for expressing his need for information; i.e. was he given the chance to put *questions*?

(6) Was the patient's *need for information* adequately *attended to* and did this happen independently of patient characteristics?

*Results*

The visit on the medical psychosomatic ward lasts a mean time of 6.7 min; pre- and post-visit discussions take up approximately another 3 min. Throughout the period under investigation visit duration was twice to three times as long as duration on traditional wards. This increase in duration goes along with an increase in utterances: 97 sentences per visit (44 per patient) are spoken on the Ulm ward in relation to 43 sentences (13 per patient) on the wards examined in the Marburg studies. The total amount of utterances has doubled. The patient at Ulm utters three times as many sentences as patients in the Marburg studies. The comparison between Ulm and Hamburg for which patient samples were matched offers the following more detailed observation: speech activity of doctors is equally high for both wards in absolute terms. Patients in Ulm are 2½ times more active verbally than patients in Hamburg [*Safian* et al., 1982]. The distribution of speech activity has shifted clearly in favour of the patient; this is due in particular to the participation of other team members being kept to a minimum (fig. 2). The doctor directs himself almost exclusively to the patient. On the traditional ward such 'patient-centered speech' [*Jährig and Koch,* 1982] accounts for only 30% of doctor's total speech time (fig. 3). Patients on the Ulm ward are offered a little more information by the doctor: at Ulm 15.8 sentences per visit contain illness-related information, on the traditional wards examined in the Marburg studies 12.6 sentences contain

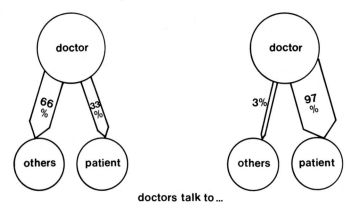

Fig. 3. Direction in which doctors talk during rounds.

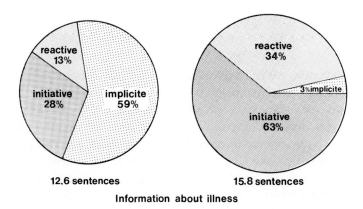

Information about illness

Fig. 4. Quantity and modes of information given to patients during rounds.

such information. The amount of information given does not increase pro-portionally with visit duration or speech activity, however. Directing infor-mation at the patient seems to require an extensive conversation. On the wards under investigation in the Marburg studies information is mostly given *indirectly* ['implicit mode of information', *Begemann-Deppe*, 1978], i.e. patients have to extract information about their illness from conver-sations going on about them in the team. In Ulm information is almost exclusively given *directly:* the doctor either offers it spontaneously, on his own initiative ('initiative mode of information'), or he reacts to a patient's request for information ('reactive mode of information') (fig. 4). The con-

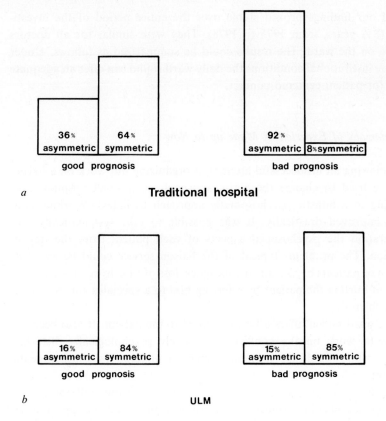

good prognosis      bad prognosis

*a*      **Traditional hospital**

good prognosis      bad prognosis

*b*      **ULM**

*Fig. 5a, b.* Quality of answers doctors give if patients put questions about their illness during rounds.

tent of information given to patients relates to psychosocial themes more often on the Ulm ward than on the Hamburg ward [*Safian* et al., 1982].

On the Ulm ward patients express a need for information more often. They ask three *questions* per visit, whereas patients on all other wards ask only one question per visit.

*Siegrist* [1976, 1978] reports that doctors answered the questions of patients with an unfavourable prognosis either not at all or evasively (in 92% of the cases investigated). Such an 'asymmetrical reaction' was more rare at Ulm (20% of all cases). Notably no difference was made between patients with favourable and unfavourable prognoses (fig. 5a, b).

All our findings proved stable over the entire period of the investigation (3½ years, from 1975 to 1978). They were similar for all doctors working on the ward. The results could be summarized as follows. Under adequate institutional conditions the daily ward round can offer an adequate setting for patient-centered contact.

## Summary of Experiences Made up to Now

Following an unsuccessful attempt at organizing our work on a liaison basis, we tried to change the entire approach on a small hospital ward according to a holistic psychosomatic approach to illness. Working conditions improved drastically. It was possible to take systematically into consideration the psychosocial aspects of each patient from the day of admission. The problems typical of the liaison service could be avoided: selection of patients by untrained colleagues, loss of time by referral, and the danger of hurting the patient by referring him to a specialist for 'psychological problems'.

The ward milieu offers a lot of support to the patient. It also becomes possible to work on the conflicts of severely psychologically disturbed patients, who would not normally agree to undergo psychotherapeutic treatment.

For us as clinical psychosomaticists – also for visiting colleagues from other departments of the centre – the ward presented excellent opportunities for further training. It also offered a working climate in which we could find our identity as psychosomaticists (just as some physicians might find their identity in their clinical laboratory). For our colleagues in the centre, the psychosomatic approach took on more distinct features and found more widespread acceptance.

A ward concept such as ours presents ample opportunities for research and the development of comprehensive therapy concepts for patients with such conditions as anorexia nervosa or asthma bronchiale for example. In most cases we were unable to solve the problems of long-term psychotherapeutic aftercare. This was due partly to the fact that patients came from a large area.

Today we believe – as indeed do most psychosomaticists in the Federal Republic of Germany – that a ward ought to be the nucleus of every independent psychosomatic department. On that basis it is much easier to provide a liaison service for other hospital divisions. We see ourselves as psychosomaticists with a strong link with internal medicine. Under advantageous conditions, such as the ones described, it ought to be possible to integrate the psychosomatic approach into medical patient care. An integration on the level of routine care requires intensive cooperation with supervisors. In our case it paid off to work together with an experienced internal specialist as supervisor [*Köhle and Kubanek*, 1981].

For the institutionalization of psychosomatic medicine, it seems important to me that the work on such a ward should take on a distinct 'Gestalt'. In Ulm we succeeded in interesting the general public by showing a documentary film (among other activities). The strong support lent by the general public to this ward was a great help in the struggle for 'survival' of the department when *von Uexküll* retired. This happened at a time when opponents of psychosomatic medicine had been trying to bring about considerable restrictions on the Department of Psychosomatics.

## References

Balint, E.; Norell, J.S.: Six minutes for the patient: interactions in general practice consultation. The Contributors (1973).

Begemann-Deppe, M.: Sprechverhalten und Thematisierung von Krankheitsinformation im Rahmen von Stationsvisiten; Dissertation, Freiburg i.Br. (1978).

Gaus, E.; Klingenburg, M.; Simons, C.; Westphale, C.; Köhle, K.: Die Funktion von Stationskonferenzen im Rahmen eines internistisch-psychosomatischen Stationskonzeptes. Verh. dt. Ges. inn. Med. *86:* 1487–1491 (1980).

Jährig, C.; Koch, U.: Die Arzt-Patienten-Interaktion in den internistischen Visiten eines Akutkrankenhauses; in Köhle, Raspe, Das ärztliche Gespräch während der Visite. Empirische Untersuchungen (Urban & Schwarzenberg, München 1982).

Karstens, R.: Psychosomatic medicine. IV. Difficulties of integration. Psychother. Psychosom. *22:* 196–199 (1973).

Köhle, K.; Kubanek, B.: Zur Zusammenarbeit von Psychosomatikern und Internisten. Erfahrungen aus 12 Jahren; in von Uexküll, Integrierte psychosomatische Medizin, pp. 17–54 (Schattauer, Stuttgart 1981).

Köhle, K.; Simons, C.; Böck, D.; Grauhan, A.: Angewandte Psychosomatik. Die internistisch-psychosomatische Krankenstation. Ein Werkstattbericht; 2nd ed. (Rocom, Basel 1980).

Köhle, K.; Simons, C.; Scholich, B.; Schäfer, N.: Psychosomatic medicine. V. Critical theses concerning the future development of integrated psychosomatic departments. Psychother. Psychosom. *22:* 200–204 (1973).

Morgan, W.L.; Engel, G.L.: The clinical approach to the patient (Saunders, Philadelphia 1969).

Nordmeyer, J.: Formal-quantitative Aspekte der Arzt-Patient-Beziehung während der Visite; in Köhle, Raspe, Das ärztliche Gespräch während der Visite (Urban & Schwarzenberg, München 1982).

Raspe, H.-H.: Das Problem der Aufklärung und Information bei Akutkrankenhaus-patienten und seine Erforschung; Dissertation, Freiburg i.Br. (1979).

Raspe, H.H.: Visitenforschung in der Bundesrepublik: Historische Reminiszenzen und Ergebnisse formal-quantitativer Analysen; in Köhle, Raspe, Das ärztliche Gespräch während der Visite. Empirische Untersuchungen (Urban & Schwarzenberg, München 1982).

Raspe, H.H.; Nordmeyer, J.: Die Stationsarztvisite – eine verschenkte Möglichkeit? Therapiewoche *31:* 1021–1025 (1981).

Rotmann, M.: Psychosomatic medicine. II. A model of an integrated psychosomatic consultation service. Psychother. Psychosom. *22:* 189–191 (1973).

Safian, P.; Fauler, I.; Koch, U.; Jährig, C.; Köhle, K.: Inhaltliche und methodische Analyse von Visitengesprächen zweier klinischer Populationen mittels unterschied-licher Rating-Verfahren; in Köhle, Raspe, Das ärztliche Gespräch während der Visite. Empirische Untersuchungen (Urban & Schwarzenberg, München 1982).

Schüffel, W.: Psychosomatic medicine. III. Patients of the psychosomatic consultant. Psychother. Psychosom. *22:* 192–195 (1973).

Siegrist, J.: Asymmetrische Kommunikation bei klinischen Visiten. Medsche Klin. *71:* 1962–1966 (1976).

Siegrist, J.: Arbeit und Interaktion im Krankenhaus (Enke, Stuttgart 1978).

Uexküll, T. von: Psychosomatic medicine. I. Subspeciality or an integrated discipline? Psychother. Psychosom. *22:* 185–188 (1973).

Uexküll, T. von: Die Chefarztvisite als Problem. Medsche Klin. *72:* 269–276 (1977).

Weed, L.L.: Medical records, medical education, and patient care (Case Western Reserve University Press, Chicago 1971).

Westphale, C.; Köhle, K.: Visitengespräche: Gesprächssituation und Informationsver-halten. Abschlussbericht aus dem Teilprojekt B 5 des SFB 129 der Deutschen For-schungsgemeinschaft an der Universität Ulm; Unveröffentl. Manuskript, Ulm (1982).

Prof. Dr. Karl Köhle, Department of Psychosomatic Medicine,
University of Ulm, Am Hochsträss 8, D-7900 Ulm (FRG)

Adv. psychosom. Med., vol. 11, pp. 191–197 (Karger, Basel 1983)

# Psychosomatic Inpatient Therapy in West Germany

*H. Neun[a], F. Lamprecht[b], I. Lützenkirchen, G.H. Wittich[c]*

[a]Niedersächsisches Landeskrankenhaus Tiefenbrunn,
 Abteilung Psychosomatische Medizin, Rosdorf b. Göttingen (FRG);
[b]Psychosomatische Klinik, Schömberg (FRG);
[c]Psychosomatische Klinik «Kinzigtal», Gengenbach (FRG)

This section documents the resources for inpatient therapy of patients suffering from psychosomatic illness in West Germany. It is based on the results of a questionnaire designed by the authors in the framework of a DKPM (German College of Psychosomatic Medicine) study group in 1978. Information was collected from institutions considering themselves as psychosomatic hospitals or as psychosomatic departments.

The following aspects were put into consideration: (1) institutional aspects; (2) internal organisation, and (3) therapeutic concepts and postgraduate training programs for residents and staff members.

## (1) *Institutional Aspects*

Generally, the owner of the institution has to cover both building and running costs. The administration makes the working contracts with the staff. However, the patients' daily hospital and treatment costs are financed by various social insurance and health insurance companies.

There are mainly three different approaches to psychosomatic inpatient therapy in West Germany: (1) consultation services; (2) psychosomatic wards with additional consultation service offered to other departments, and (3) psychosomatic and psychotherapeutic hospitals.

### *Consultation Services* (table I)

The majority of them are placed within the framework of a university general hospital. Public organisations, usually the district government, are responsible for the financial aspects of it. These services cover the needs of

*Table I.* Consultation services for psychosomatic medicine (n=11)

| | | |
|---|---|---|
| Financing of building and running costs | public organisations | 9 |
| | nonprofit organisations | 2 |
| | private organisations | 0 |
| Financing of treatment | health insurance | 6 |
| | annuity insurance/public assistance | 1 |
| | professional and trade associations | 1 |
| | private | 1 |
| | social welfare | 1 |
| Contract of staff members as | official | 8 |
| | salaried employee | 10 |
| | consultant (freelance) | 3 |
| Service in | general hospitals | 1 |
| | psychiatric clinics | 0 |
| | internal medicine clinics | 3 |
| | other clinics | 3 |
| | university/college ('Lehrstuhl') | 3 |
| | university department | 6 |
| | research institute | 1 |
| Organised as | 'department' | 5 |
| | with outpatient clinic | 11 |
| Frequent cooperation with | other clinics (inpatient treatment) | 5 |
| | other outpatient clinics | 7 |
| | diagnostic facilities | 2 |
| | doctors (own practice) | 7 |
| | regional university clinics of psychosomatic medicine | 1 |

hospital departments as well as those of the connected outpatient clinics. There is a high incidence of cooperation with other institutions and with doctors in own practice.

Treatment costs are provided by the insurance companies or by the government as part of the social welfare program, and in a few instances by the private patient himself.

For inpatients, consultation service included, a global sum is provided, negotiated yearly by the insurance companies and the hospital administration. The same is true for outpatient clinics of the universities. For outpatient departments outside university facilities, there is no standard fee, but remuneration depends on the services rendered.

### Psychosomatic Wards with Additional Consultation Service
### Offered to Other Departments (table II)

Most of these departments are run and financed by public organisations. Nearly one-third of them do not have outpatient facilities, are not university affiliated and still at the same time have the largest number of inpatients. In most cases there are between 10 and 16 patients on a ward.

This type of inpatient treatment necessarily has to be time-limited. The average length of stay ranges from 6 to 12 weeks. Frequent cooperation with other departments and with general practitioners takes place.

*Psychosomatic and Psychotherapeutic Hospitals* (table II)

Different from the above-mentioned institutions, 17 specialised psychosomatic and psychotherapeutic hospitals are run and financed by private organisations offering a very broad range of contracts to their staff. Duties, position within the team, salary, etc., vary to a high degree and this, in turn, may influence the doctor-patient relationship. The majority of these institutions also invite part-time consultants to cooperate.

Most of these hospitals, whose bed capacity ranges from 10 to 50, have outpatient facilities as well. But there seem to be many restrictions insofar as usually just one staff member – often the medical director – gets a contract with the insurance companies; and at the same time his outpatient therapy will be restricted to one method, for instance psychoanalytic-oriented psychotherapy.

(2) *Internal Organisation* (table III)

In order to gather data concerning internal organisation of the institutions, we asked for the number and qualification of staff members, their responsibilities and aspects of team work. To give an example: one of the psychosomatic university departments represents a typical example of a *consultation service*. There are 9 doctors and clinical psychologists, the head of the department and the chief of staff. All of them spend 2 h a week on teamwork. Different to this, another psychological research institute of a university reports a much higher amount of time spent in the team.

Teamwork has not been defined in this study. Possible topics of discussion are decisions to be taken in regard to patients' admission and the therapeutic program, recruiting of new staff members and running costs. It was found that mainly doctors and psychologists decide on patients' admission and that at the same time the therapy program is proposed by the senior members of the staff. Recruiting new staff members, however, is a field in which all doctors and psychologists participate.

Hardly any influence of doctors and psychologists has been reported on financial matters.

All departments and their therapeutic team offer a combination of therapeutic approaches within a particular ward setting. The doctor/patient relation ranges around 1:7 which is considered very satisfactory.

*Table II.* Psychosomatic and psychotherapeutic hospitals (n = 17), and departments with ward and consultation services for psychosomatic medicine (n = 18)

| | | Hosp. | Dep. |
|---|---|---|---|
| Financing of building and running costs | public organisations | 3 | 13 |
| | nonprofit organisations | 2 | 3 |
| | private organisations | 12 | 2 |
| Financing of treatment | health insurance | 16 | 18 |
| | annuity insurance/public assistance | 4 | 4 |
| | professional and trade associations | 5 | 1 |
| | private | 3 | 7 |
| | social welfare | 7 | 3 |
| Contract of staff members as | official | 2 | 7 |
| | salaried employee | 17 | 18 |
| | consultant (freelance) | 7 | 2 |
| Service and wards in | general hospitals | | 4 |
| | psychiatric clinics | | 6 |
| | internal medicine clinics | | 7 |
| | other clinics | | 1 |
| | university/colleges ('Lehrstuhl') | | 8 |
| | university/departments | | 2 |
| Organized as | 'hospital' | 17 | |
| | 'department' | | 18 |
| | 'independent clinic' | | 3 |
| | with outpatient facilities | 14 | 9 |
| | without outpatient facilities* | 3 | 7 |
| Frequent cooperation with | other clinics (inpatient treatment) | 11 | 11 |
| | other outpatient clinics | 6 | 6 |
| | diagnostic facilities | 6 | 6 |
| | doctors (own practice) | 16 | 16 |
| | regional university clinics of psychosomatic medicine | 0 | 0 |
| | social psychiatric services | 1 | 1 |
| | employment office | 7 | 7 |
| | counseling services (education) | 2 | 2 |
| | other institutions | 5 | 5 |

Concerning psychosomatic and psychotherapeutic hospitals, an interesting characteristic of the staff attitude towards teamwork appears to be the answer: all activities carried out by the staff are considered team work.

## (3) *Basic Concepts* (table IV)

The majority of consultation services and almost all departments and hospitals considered the psychoanalytic theory to be the conceptual basis of

*Table II.* (continued)

| Capacity (Hosp.) | 1 | 2 | 3 | 4 | 5 | 6 | 7 | 8 | 9 | 10 | 11 | 12 | 13 | 14 | 15 | 16 | 17 |
|---|---|---|---|---|---|---|---|---|---|---|---|---|---|---|---|---|---|
| Number of patients per ward | 20 | 21 | ? | 25 | ? 20 | | 20 | 10 | 19 | ? 24 | | 21 | 50 | 10 | 11 12 16 22 | 25 27 | 20 |
| Total number of patients | 115 | 21* | 65 | 187 | 50 | 80 | 220 | 21 | 225* | 95 | 24* | 208 | 250 | 102* | 176* | 130* | 200 |

Total number of patients in
 University departments        24
 Nonuniversity departments   2145
 Privately financed clinics   1565

Average length of treatment   < 6         weeks in 10 institutions
                              6–12       weeks in 13 institutions
               more than    12 weeks in  4 institutions

| Capacity (Dep.) | 1 | 2 | 3 | 4 | 5 | 6 | 7 | 8 | 9 | 10 | 11 | 12 | 13 | 14 | 15 | 16 | 17 | 18 |
|---|---|---|---|---|---|---|---|---|---|---|---|---|---|---|---|---|---|---|
| Number of wards | 1 | 1 | 2 | 2 | 1 | 1 | 1 | 3 | 1 | 1 | 1 | 1 | 3 | 3 | 3 | 1 | 1 | 1 |
| Number of patients per ward | 15 | 10 | 16 | 45 | 20 | 10 | 15 | 16 | 15 | 34 | 11 | 10 | 13 24 22 | 12 20 | 12 | 15 | 15 | 24 |
| Total number of patients | 15 | 10 | 100* | 60 | 16 | 10 | 15 | 44 | 15 | 34* | 11 | 10 | 50 | 48 | 54* | 15 | 15 | 24 |

Total number of patients in
 University departments        243
 Nonuniversity departments     213

Average length of treatment   < 6         weeks in 4 institutions
                              6–12       weeks in 9 institutions
               more than    12 weeks in 5 institutions

their approach; only a few mention an integrative psychosomatic concept. Consultation services differ from the latter as to the idea what should be considered to be the most effective factor in treatment. They emphasise the value either of a single method or of a combination of methods applied. The questionnaires of hospitals and departments on the other hand indicate that a combination of the ward setting and the patient's relationship with the staff are thought to be the most effective factors. These attitudes seem to illustrate the different ways of applying the psychoanalytic concept in practice.

Table III. Consultation services for psychosomatic medicine (n = 11)

| | Number in each service | | | | | | | | | | |
|---|---|---|---|---|---|---|---|---|---|---|---|
| | 1 | 2 | 3 | 4 | 5 | 6 | 7 | 8 | 9 | 10 | 11 |
| *Staff members* | | | | | | | | | | | |
| Doctors and psychologists | 5 | 17 | 4 | 11 | 4 | 3 | 7 | 9 | 10 | 1 | 5 |
| Social workers | 1* | – | – | – | – | 3 | 4 | – | – | – | – |
| Physical therapists | 1* | – | – | – | – | 3 | – | – | – | – | – |
| *Directorial functions (in contract)* | | | | | | | | | | | |
| Department heads | 1 | 4 | 1 | – | 1 | – | 1 | 1 | 1 | – | 1 |
| Deputy heads | 1 | – | 1 | – | 1 | – | 1 | 1 | 1 | – | – |
| *Teamwork (hours a week)* | | | | | | | | | | | average |
| Medical heads | 9 | | 10 | 11 | | | 7 | 2 | 7 | | 2–11 h |
| Other staff | | | 6 | 17 | | 7 | | 2 | 7 | | 7  2–17 h |

*The therapeutic unit defined as* Department, 7; ward, –; other, 1

| | Adminis-tration | Medical heads | Doctors and psychologists | Total staff |
|---|---|---|---|---|
| *Final authority regarding* | | | | |
| Patient's admission | – | – | 5 | 2 |
| Program of therapy | – | 5 | 3 | 4 |
| Employment of staff | 3 | – | 4 | 2 |
| Running costs | 5 | – | 3 | 2 |

* Part time.

Correspondingly, a combined treatment program is favored by hospitals and departments. As a rule, this combination includes a medical approach, social therapy and psychotherapy.

There is also a considerable difference as to the use of postclinical treatment. Consultation services offer postclinical treatments in their own outpatient facilities. Departments, because of lack of outpatient facilities, rather refer the discharged patients to practicing psychotherapists. Hospitals, on the other hand, rarely refer to practicing psychotherapists but rather offer a follow-up inpatient treatment according to the principles of interval therapy.

In spite of the general accepted basis of a psychoanalytic approach, views in regard to supervision seem to differ. If there is any supervision in consultation services at all, it is carried out in various ways by different persons. In departments, supervision is often practiced by the head of the

*Table IV*. Theoretical orientation in institutions for psychosomatic medicine

|  | I) Consultation services (n = 11) | II) Departments (n = 18) | III) Hospitals (n = 17) |
|---|---|---|---|
| Staff supervision by (diagnosis of staff conflicts and group dynamics) |  |  |  |
| None | 4 | 2 | 1 |
| The entire staff | 5 | 7 (3) | 9 (2) |
| Departmental head | 3 | 7 | 3 (3) |
| Head physician | 1 | 6 (1) | 3 |
| Consultant (part time) | 3 | 2 | 7 (3) |
| Further training (entitled to offer) |  |  |  |
| Psychotherapy | 4 | 14 | 15 |
| Psychoanalysis | 3 | 3 | 5 |
| In cooperation with a psychoanalytic institute | 3 | 12 | 11 |

(I) = This type only.

department or senior staff members, depending on the structure of the institution; therefore, these supervisors are in many cases members of the team.

As to psychosomatic hospitals, there seem to be two different views and practice: either supervision is carried out by the entire staff or by qualified part-time consultants not otherwise affiliated to the institution.

Information reported on further training confirms the predominant role of psychoanalysis. Most of the departments and clinics cooperate closely with a psychoanalytic institute offering a systematic long-range training, the curriculum and requirements being set both by the medical association and international psychoanalytic societies. A certificate is given upon completion of the psychoanalytic training program.

*Final Considerations*

Further information about psychosomatic inpatient therapy is necessary. Much effort should be put into improving working conditions as well as into establishing and promoting training and supervision programs. There is a need for further research in regard to institutional conditions as prerequisites of inpatient psychosomatic and psychotherapeutic therapy.

H. Neun, MD, Niedersächsisches Landeskrankenhaus Tiefenbrunn,
Abteilung Psychosomatische Medizin, D-3405 Rosdorf b. Göttingen (FRG)

Adv. psychosom. Med., vol. 11, pp. 198–204 (Karger, Basel 1983)

# Balint Group Work and Final Conclusions[1]

*Hubert Speidel*

Department of Psychosomatics, University Hospital Eppendorf, Hamburg, FRG

## Balint Group Work

In the immediate post-war period *Michael Balint* was one of the first psychoanalysts to come and work in Germany. His influence had a decisive catalysing effect in reviving German psychoanalysis. Concurrently *Balint's* method of training general practitioners in psychoanalytically oriented groups has become very popular [*Luban-Plozza*, 1974]; many regard this as the best way of providing practitioners with insight into psychosomatic medicine. Thus, liaison medicine in West Germany is largely based on Balint group work.

The aim of a Balint group is to help the general practitioner, and not the psychotherapist, to recognise and understand the psychological aspects of his patient's disease, so that within the framework of his normal practice he feels competent to offer psychotherapeutic support. The focus of interest is the relationship between doctor and patient, and how these two can work together to solve the patient's problem. The setting is as follows: The group and its leader meet, over a span of 3 years or more, once a week for 1.5–2 h, with the express purpose of discussing cases which the group members have come across in their own practices. A 'case' in this sense is not just the patient, but includes the doctor as well, with the transference and countertransference processes involved in their relationship to one another. The point of the discussion is to help the doctor to understand and possibly modify his own attitudes by indirectly increasing his self-awareness; as soon as he has gained a better insight into his own unconscious and preconscious reactions, he is in a much better position to perceive the psychological and social pressures which are

---

[1] Translated by Dr. *Jane Wiebel*.

troubling his patient. Instead of going into a single case at great length and in great detail, as would normally be the case in a psychotherapeutic supervision session, the group concentrates on interpreting particular episodes or situations which have raised problems for the doctor during his daily routine (flash technique). The members of the group all have an important role to play; collectively they act as a prism [*Loch*, 1972], each contributing his own reaction and so highlighting different aspects of either the patient's or the doctor's behaviour in the episode under scrutiny. The group leader can then take up this material and help to interpret it. The longer the group has been established, the easier this becomes, as the members soon come to recognise their own and one another's reactions and responses. The way in which the group leader behaves serves as a model for the doctor in his relationship to his patient. He intervenes in the discussion only moderately, behaves as an equal and not as an authority, and is careful to restrict his interpretations and confrontations to a level which keeps in check regressive tendencies in the group [*Balint*, 1964; *Speidel*, 1975, 1977].

In the past 10 years Balint group work has extended beyond the sphere of the general practitioner, and is now gradually spreading into hospitals and institutions [*Drees*, 1980; *Köhle*, 1981]. This has meant that some modifications have had to be made in the technique, as patients in hospital are faced with quite different problems; many of them already have long histories as patients and are being cared for by specialists, they are often unable to consider the psychological side of their illness, and they are frequently treated by doctors who they did not personally choose. In cases of this kind the illness has become 'organised' [*Balint*, 1964], in that the patient clings to certain pseudoexplanations on the organic level for his illness, and the illness is often more severe. The relationship between the patient and his doctor is often just a temporary affair, and no single doctor can take responsibility for curing him. Group work in a hospital setting comes closest to the classical Balint group when those taking part are all doctors from different departments who, as in the classical setting, do not know each other's patients. Usually, however, another setting is chosen, involving a group leader and the nursing staff or the doctors or the whole team in a single department. In this case most of the participants know the patients being discussed, and this means that the emphasis in the group work changes. While listening to another member's account of how he fared with a specific patient, each member can draw on his own experience and response to the same patient. Another topic, which does not come up in the classical setting, is how the members of the team get on with one another on the ward, and this has to be discussed in the group as well. There are three possible ways of structuring this type of group work:

(1) The interactional problems within the team are firmly excluded,

and group work takes place as a modified form of Balint group work. This method is only viable where the team functions relatively smoothly, and the problems which crop up do not impinge on group discussions on patients.

(2) Depending on the case under discussion, the group functions either as a Balint group or as a counselling forum for the team. In practice it is difficult to keep these two types apart, and switching from one to the other is tricky.

(3) If the group members find it so difficult to cooperate with one another on the ward that the patients suffer as a consequence, it is worth introducing an indirect form of liaison medicine, i.e. a job-oriented self-awareness group comprising the entire team. This is of course only feasible if all agree to take part [*Ramb and Speidel*, 1977; *Speidel*, 1975, 1977].

To illustrate this point, a brief description of one such group is given. I had arranged to run a Balint group for the whole team working in a department for child and juvenile psychiatry, but it soon became obvious that the most pressing problems were not to be found between staff and patients, but among the staff themselves. We therefore decided to meet as a group with a different purpose in mind; the topic was now how each member of the staff saw himself or herself in relation to the others on the ward, and discussion centred on all the emotional and communication problems which had arisen (job-oriented self-awareness group). It was particularly lucky that the head of department, who was relatively new, was keen to get the group working. He suffered most from the tensions in the team he had taken over, and was therefore personally highly motivated. Apart from one or two nurses, all the staff joined in (doctors, psychologists, teachers and nurses). After 3 years the staff could work so cooperatively together that group work could be brought to a close. The feuds between rival professional groups and factions had ceased, and instead the team was now able to discuss its differences in a sober, constructive and tolerant manner. All the participants agreed that the patients and their families profited directly from this improved atmosphere, and the staff members stressed that they themselves now got more satisfaction out of their work. A follow-up 1.5 years later showed that this style of working which had been learned in the group was still functioning well, although some members had left to continue their training or set up in private practice, and had been replaced by newcomers [*Ramb and Speidel*, 1977; *Speidel*, 1977, and in press].

Drawing on this and related experiences, we can divide group work up into various categories to suit different situations: If the aim is above all to give hospital staff better insight into their own behaviour, so that they can work better as a team, the setting should be a group consisting of all staff members, and the topic should be the members' reactions and responses to one another within the framework of the ward (a job-oriented self-awareness group). In this type of group it is important that the members, and especially the head of the department, are really interested in improving matters and are sufficiently motivated to keep attending. If on the other hand the point is to help each individual member to improve his competence in psychological medicine, so that he can care for his patients better, then the classical Balint group is a most effective setting, with one important modification; if the group consists of therapists who all work in different departments, it is important to include their relationships to the rest of the medical staff on the wards in the group discussion [*Speidel*, in press].

These modified forms of Balint group work have proved quite flexible and can be adapted to accommodate other needs, for instance those of students in training. During the final stage of their medical training, students in West Germany are required to do practical work in hospital (known as the 'practical year'). This means that they work in a surgical and clinical department, and in another department of their own choice; between these blocks they have a month off to pursue their studies [*Meyer*, 1979]. Several of the university psychosomatic departments, including the one in Hamburg, have set up 'junior' Balint groups to help the students cope with these new demands [*Luban-Plozza*, 1979]. In these groups discussion centres round how to build up a good relationship to the patients, a problem which many of the students find hard to solve, and around their own feelings of inferiority and superfluity on the wards, their unsatisfactory status which prevents them from taking over any real responsibility, and their often strained relationships with the medical staff, the discrepancy they feel between their clinical inexperience and their personal psychosocial ability, and the narcissistic problems which arise out of this frustrating situation. The junior Balint groups continue to meet throughout the entire 'practical year'.

To illustrate another field in which modified Balint group work can pay dividends, I should like to mention the group I run for the staff working in liaison medicine in the Department of Medical Psychology in Hamburg University. Most of those taking part are clinical psychologists involved in the care of cancer patients in a tumour centre, as part of a long-term project. The supervision this work requires is offered in the form of a Balint group. The problems which have come up for discussion include, especially at first, general inexperience in dealing with terminal patients, the psychologists' feeling of inferiority compared with their doctor colleagues on the ward, various conflict situations which prove difficult to handle, and personal disagreements amongst the staff. Because of numerous commitments and demands on their time – research, teaching students, administrative duties – it was often hard for the members to find time to attend our sessions. The work in the group has proved fruitful in several respects; it has helped to stabilise the psychologists' self-esteem, enabled them to work out new and better ways of organising their work on the wards and encouraged them to lay down reasonable limits for their involvement with the patients [*Speidel*, in press].

## Out-Patient Setting

Surprisingly enough there is very little liaison work being done in out-patient settings in West Germany, although this would seem the most sensible area in which to set it up, with a view to giving the patient proper care right from the start. In Hamburg we have been trying out a new scheme for the past year; one of our colleagues from the psychosomatic department spends one full morning a week in the clinical out-patient department, seeing all the patients her clinical colleagues think need her help, and giving patients and doctors advice. The results so far are encouraging. The patients with psychosocial problems are diagnosed before any treatment gets under way, and since the case can be discussed immediately with the clinicians, no time is lost in organising the help necessary. Another advantage is that the out-patient doctors themselves become more competent in diagnosing psychological and social problems.

## General Final Remarks

To summarise, Balint group work and allied forms of it are used widely in West Germany. The term liaison medicine itself is unknown, except to a few insiders. If we restrict the term to the sense in which it is applied in the USA [*Pasnau*, 1975; *Greenhill*, 1977; *Speidel*, 1980], there is very little liaison medicine here at all [*Speidel*, in press]. If, however, we define the work in terms of its purpose, then Balint group work and its variations are a form of liaison medicine which has developed here quite naturally and is in that sense characteristic. In fact, liaison medicine in any form has to contend with all kinds of difficulties:

(1) Many of the elderly doctors who are now in influential positions had an exclusively scientific training, and are more or less deeply prejudiced against psychology.

(2) Power struggles and arguments about who has the last say are just as rife here as in the USA, and often mar attempts to get clinicians and psychologists to cooperate with one another.

(3) There is a genuine shortage of properly qualified personnel, and this naturally limits expansion. On the other hand, this fact is often used as a defensive rationalisation to justify the lack of progress in liaison medicine.

(4) The psychosomatic departments do not have unlimited resources, and since they are responsible for training students and offering an advisory

service for the entire hospital, there is often no time or energy left for liaison medicine.

(5) This argument tends to be used as a defense. The real reason is that those working in psychosomatics may be apprehensive about getting involved in clinical medicine. This is certainly true of the psychologists, whose training rarely brings them in contact with hospital patients [Speidel, 1982], but it applies equally to those doctors who have had psychotherapeutic training and are more or less unwilling to remain in touch with their clinical colleagues. In fact, the longer their psychotherapeutic training lasts, the more they tend to move away from the field of organic medicine.

(6) Both organic medicine and psychiatry in West Germany look back on an exclusively scientific tradition, which continues to exert a negative influence. A clinician, for instance, who takes part in post-graduate training, is not required to know anything about psychology at all, a highly anachronistic state of affairs which pushes psychosomatics into the background and instead stresses other, purely scientific aspects of medicine [Speidel, 1981]. Some universities have even refused to establish chairs for psychosomatics/psychotherapy, although the new regulations demand that this subject be offered to all medical students [Meyer, 1979]. As a result some well-established universities like Bonn and Munich have remained backward. Since the new regulations have laid down that psychosomatics/psychotherapy is now obligatory before the student can graduate, there is bound to be a change for the better in liaison medicine, and it seems likely that in the next few years we will see a lot of experimenting on how clinicians and psychologists can pool their knowledge more effectively. By the time the students of today have become the heads of department of tomorrow, the situation will have changed for the better.

## References

Balint, M.: The doctor, his patient and the illness (Pitmen Medical Publishing Co., London 1964).

Drees, A.: Balint-Gruppen in Institutionen. Fortschr. Med. *98:* 1554–1556 (1980).

Greenhill, M.H.: The development of liaison program; in Usdin, Psychiatric medicine, pp. 115–193 (Brunner, New York 1977).

Köhle, K.: Klinisch-psychosomatische Krankenstationen; in Uexküll, Lehrbuch der Psychosomatischen Medizin; 2nd ed., pp. 299–326 (Urban & Schwarzenberg, München 1981).

Loch, W.: Psychotherapeutische Behandlung psychosomatischer Erkrankungen; in Loch,

Zur Theorie, Technik und Therapie der Psychoanalyse, pp. 269–282 (Fischer, Frankfurt a.M. 1972).

Luban-Plozza, B.: Praxis der Balint-Gruppen. Beziehungsdiagnostik und Therapie (Lehmann, München 1974).

Luban-Plozza, B.: Zehn Jahre Balint-Gruppen mit Studenten. Dt. Ärztebl. *33:* 585–590 (1979).

Meyer, A.-E.: German developments in teaching psychosomatic and psychotherapy to medical students. Psychother. Psychosom. *31:* 75–80 (1979).

Pasnau, R.D., ed.: Consultation-liaison psychiatry (Grune & Stratton, New York 1975).

Ramb, W.; Speidel, H.: Teamgruppen-Arbeit an einer psychiatrisch-psychosomatischen Klinik für Kinder und Jugendliche. Therapiewoche *27:* 7030–7036 (1977).

Speidel, H.: Die Balint-Gruppe. Möglichkeiten zum kontrollierten Erwerb psychosomatischen Verständnisses. Therapiewoche *25:* 3696–3700 (1975).

Speidel, H.: Die Balint-Gruppe. Voraussetzungen, Theorie und Methodik. Therapiewoche *27:* 6946–6961 (1977).

Speidel, H.: Konsultations- und Liaisondienste. Verh. dt. Ges. inn. Med. *86:* 1506 (1980).

Speidel, H.: Probleme der Zusammenarbeit zwischen Organmedizin und psychosomatischer Medizin. Therapiewoche *31:* 980–986 (1981).

Speidel, H.: Relation between psychiatrists and colleagues in parapsychiatric professions; in Lopez-Ibor Aliño, Training and education in psychiatry (Toray, Barcelona, in press).

Prof. Dr. med. H. Speidel, Professor of Psychosomatics and Psychotherapy,
University of Hamburg, Eppendorf Hospital, Martinistrasse 52,
D–2000 Hamburg 20 (FRG)

Adv. psychosom. Med., vol. 11, pp. 205–209 (Karger, Basel 1983)

# International Comparisons: Concluding Remarks

*Geoffrey Lloyd*

Consultant Psychiatrist, Royal Infirmary, Edinburgh, Scotland

The breadth of activities described in this volume testifies to the changing role of psychiatry in many different countries and in widely varying cultural settings. The general hospital is now firmly established as a legitimate area for psychiatric practice and research. Recognition of the high prevalence of psychiatric illness among medical patients and the adverse effects it confers on general health has provided a foundation for psychiatry to develop within general medicine. This opportunity has been seized by many, being particularly encouraged by those who see liaison psychiatry as offering a means of salvation for psychiatry's image as a medical discipline [*Hackett*, 1977; *Moore*, 1978; *Eisenberg*, 1979]. From a diagnostic viewpoint, the net has been cast far beyond the traditional view of madness [*Shepherd*, 1977], thereby opening up new approaches to the management of medical patients with psychosocial problems.

But progress has not always been smooth and several factors have hindered psychiatry's expansion. At a time when many countries are facing unfamiliar economic pressures it is opportune to consider some of these barriers and to take stock of psychiatry's contribution to other medical specialties. Future developments should be based on rational decisions made in the light of clinical research and evaluative studies; uncontrolled expansion might again lead to cynicism on the part of physicians and other professional groups. Decisions also need to be taken with reference to the role of psychiatry in general as there is clear evidence that the specialty is going through another period of anguish over its viability.

## Lack of Resources

In countries where there are relatively few psychiatrists, therapeutic efforts have been concentrated on the most conspicuous forms of mental illness, the functional psychoses and the organic mental disorders. Treatment has been undertaken in antiquated mental hospitals, often far removed from large conurbations and university hospitals. This has perpetuated the alienation of psychiatry from general medicine with the consequence that psychiatrists have made little contribution to the management of medical patients. The situation is typified by Dr. *Ishikawa's* account in which he claims that the interest of orthodox Japanese psychiatrists in treating schizophrenia and depression has been associated with lack of enthusiasm for liaison and consultation work. As a result, general physicians and other specialists have become involved in the psychosomatic aspects of medicine. This greater involvement on the part of physicians is a trend which can only be welcomed but it is regrettable that it has come about by neglect.

It is no coincidence that liaison psychiatry has flourished most vigorously in the United States where there are more psychiatrists per head of population than in any other country. In addition to the legacy of psychosomatic medicine, the greater availability of American psychiatrists has enabled close integration with general medicine to develop and it has probably contributed to the high referral rates which are usually reported from American hospitals [*Lloyd*, 1980]. The development and current status of liaison psychiatry in the United States are clearly outlined in the chapters by Drs. *Leigh* and *Oken*. While acknowledging that there is no formula to define the number of psychiatrists required in each hospital Dr. *Oken* claims that ideally every clinical specialty should be covered. To achieve this in a manner which permits close liaison rather than consultation large numbers of psychiatrists are needed, both trained staff and trainees. This aspiration is achieved in some hospitals [*Hackett*, 1978] but elsewhere it will remain a pipe dream for the foreseeable future. This is particularly so for developing countries where difficult decisions have to be taken concerning the deployment of scarce medical personnel. Modelling facilities on those established in leading American hospitals is clearly inappropriate and the participation of psychiatrists in liaison rounds may not be universally suitable, nor would physicians necessarily welcome this type of psychiatric integration. Where there are shortages of staff and facilities it will be preferable for psychiatry to provide an effective consultation service before liaison is attempted.

*Resistances*

Much has been written concerning the various resistances to the expansion of liaison services. Many of these are financial and even in affluent societies departments of liaison psychiatry have to struggle for funds. The liaison psychiatrist's potential in bridging the behavioural and biological facets of medicine has rightly been stressed and it follows that the strength of the bridge depends on the adequacy of the support on either side.

The views of the medical profession towards psychiatry reflect the cultural attitudes of the society in which the doctor works. A psychological explanation of symptoms and a psychological approach to treatment are not widely accepted in some countries whereas in other cultures psychological theories have made considerable impact on popular thinking and on the medical profession. Western culture generally permits more expression and differentiation of emotional states than do traditional cultures where distress is still likely to be expressed in somatic terms [*Leff*, 1981]. Even so, reports from British and American hospitals indicate that physicians fail to recognise psychiatric morbidity in many of their patients [*Maguire* et al., 1974; *Moffic and Paykel*, 1975]. These patients, therefore, do not receive all the treatment they require and are not referred to psychiatrists. When psychiatric morbidity is recognised referral may not occur because of the physicians' dissatisfaction with the psychiatric services or antipathy towards psychiatry [*Mezey and Kellett*, 1971; *Steinberg* et al., 1980].

Where physicians and surgeons hold favourable views of psychiatry's contribution to medicine liaison-psychiatry will develop. There also needs to be encouragement from other psychiatrists so that posts can be created and funds set aside for supporting staff and facilities. Below a critical level of staffing psychiatry will make little impact within the general hospital. Lack of available beds for in-patients hampers developments in many hospitals. Dr. *Kohle's* experiences in Ulm highlight this problem; it is pertinent that he considers the ward should be the nucleus of an independent psychosomatic department and that this facility made it easier to provide a liaison service elsewhere in the hospital.

*Defining the Psychiatrist's Role*

An important question which will need to be considered in the near future is who is the most appropriate person to treat emotional problems in the medically ill. Good clinical practice has always involved attention to the emotional as well as the physical aspects of illness and there are dangers in splitting the patient's management between different doctors. The detailed contributions from West Germany are especially interesting in this context in that they report developments which are not reflected in many other countries. Psychosomatic medicine appears to have considerable relevance in West German hospitals and it is clear that the concept of psychosomatic illness has been retained, in contrast to other countries where the term has largely been abandoned [Lloyd, 1983]. The practice of psychosomatic medicine is in the hands of physicians who have also trained in psychoanalysis; the orientation of treatment is therefore psychodynamic. These psychosomatic units have often developed within departments of medicine being independent from general psychiatry and not being concerned with the treatment of the common psychiatric problems such as depressive illness, schizophrenia, alcoholism and organic brain syndromes. In this sense they assemble the Rochester model developed by Engel and Romano [Engel, 1967] but differ from the more typical liaison services which have been established elsewhere.

Many would regard this approach as controversial and consider it essential that anyone treating the emotional complications of physical illness should have received a thorough grounding in general psychiatry and not merely in psychoanalysis. Nevertheless, the German model allows clinical care to be retained by one physician and it permits unique opportunities to measure the benefits of psychotherapy in the management of physically ill patients.

Other professional groups are claiming increasing expertise in the management of mental illness and Shepherd [1982] has stressed the importance for the psychiatrist to define his own function if he is to justify his status. This has particular relevance to liaison-psychiatry which at times appears to be expanding before a secure foundation has been established. The psychiatrist is on safest ground when he is concerned with the recognition and treatment of primary psychiatric illness, whether this accompanies physical illness or is presenting with a somatic façade. He is not so secure when he assumes a prophylactic role and attempts to allay conflicts and prevent the deterioration of clinical care by mediating between patients and staff. Nor is the psychiatric treatment of emotional reactions or poor adjustment to illness firmly established. These are areas of potential benefit but they need careful evaluation and should not become the fulcrum upon which rests the future of liaison psychiatry.

*References*

Eisenberg, L.: Interfaces between medicine and psychiatry. Compreh. Psychiat. *20:* 1–14 (1979).

Engel, G.L.: Medical education and the psychosomatic approach: a report on the Rochester experience 1946–1966. J. psychosom. Res. *11:* 77–85 (1967).

Hackett, T.P.: The psychiatrist: in the mainstream or on the banks of medicine? Am. J. Psychiat. *134:* 432–434 (1977).

Hackett, T.P.: Beginnings: liaison psychiatry in a general hospital; in Hackett, Cassem, Handbook of general hospital psychiatry, pp. 1–14 (Mosby, St. Louis 1978).

Leff, J.: Psychiatry around the globe: a transcultural view (Dekker, New York 1981).

Lloyd, G.G.: Liaison psychiatry from a British perspective. Gen. Hosp. Psychiat. *2:* 46–51 (1980).

Lloyd, G.G.: Liaison psychiatry; in Hill, Murray, Thorley, Essentials of postgraduate psychiatry; 2nd ed. (Academic Press, London, in press, 1983).

Maguire, G.P.; Julier, D.L.; Hawton, K.E.; Bancroft, J.H.J.: Psychiatric morbidity and referral on two general medical wards. Br. med. J. *i:* 268–270 (1974).

Mezey, A.G.; Kellett, J.M.: Reasons against referral to the psychiatrist. Post-grad. med. J. *47:* 315–319 (1971).

Moffic, H.S.; Paykel, E.S.: Depression in medical inpatients. Br. J. Psychiat. *126:* 346–353 (1975).

Moore, G.L.: The adult psychiatrist in the medical environment. Am. J. Psychiat. *135:* 413–419 (1978).

Shepherd, M.: The extent of mental disorder: beyond the layman's madness. Can. psychiat. Ass. J. *21:* 401–409 (1977).

Shepherd, M.: Who should treat mental disorders? Lancet *i:* 1173–1175 (1982).

Steinberg, H.; Torem, M.; Saraway, S.M.: An analysis of physician resistance to psychiatric consultations. Archs gen. Psychiat. *37:* 1007–1012 (1980).

G. Lloyd, Consultant Psychiatrist, Royal Infirmary,
Edinburgh EH3 9YW (Scotland)

# Subject Index